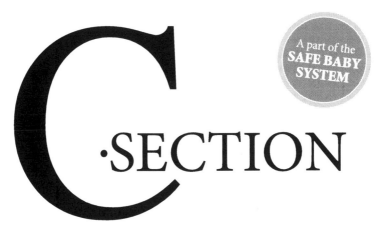

A part of the
**SAFE BABY
SYSTEM**

C·SECTION

How to **Avoid, Prepare for** and **Recover from** Your **Cesarean**

Mark Zakowski, MD

Quantum Birthing, LLC
Yorba Linda, CA

C-Section: How To Avoid, Prepare For And Recover From Your Cesarean
by Mark Zakowski MD

Publisher:
Quantum Birthing, LLC
20001 Canyon Dr.
Yorba Linda CA 92886
714-455-2992

ISBN: 978-0-9832067-1-2

Cover design: Raoul Pascual
Interior layout: Nick Zelinger

Printed in the United States of America

COMPANIES, ORGANIZATIONS, INSTITUTIONS, AND INDUSTRY PUBLICATIONS:
Quantity discounts are available on bulk purchases of this book for reselling, educational purposes, subscription incentives, gifts, sponsorship, or fundraising. Special books or book excerpts can also be created to fit specific needs such as private labeling with your logo on the cover and a message from a VIP printed inside. For more information, please contact our Special Sales Department at Quantum Birthing, LLC.

A NOTE TO READERS

The author has personally helped over 24,000 women give birth and has been Chief of OB Anesthesia for over 110,000 deliveries. The case studies in this book are generally based upon the author's considerable personal experience. In order to protect the privacy of the individuals involved, all such case studies are fictional composites of multiple situations, persons and outcomes. All names, locations and facts are the product of the author's imagination, and any resemblance to actual persons is entirely coincidental. Although real locations are mentioned, all are used fictitiously.

EDUCATIONAL ONLY

CHANGES

My book is dedicated to the tens of thousands of women giving birth who have taught me so much and who allowed me to help them in their moments of need.

I also dedicate this book to my family—to my wonderful wife and great children, and my loyal four-legged companions Harry and Tup. They inspired and encouraged me to continue, even at 1 AM.

In memoriam, to my mother, who taught me the value of education and life.

TABLE OF CONTENTS

Acknowledgements

I would like to acknowledge all my patients and colleagues—doctors, nurses, midwives and doulas. In particular, my lifelong teacher, friend and mentor Professor Sivam Ramanathan MD, Julian Gold MD, Co-Chief Department of Anesthesiology for his support and encouragement of my independent project over the last few years, ... everyone who has helped to read and re-edit the book including Rebecca, Yolande, Stephanie, Michael, Joe, Alicia, Susie, Dean, Gary K, Brian P, to the many experts who allowed me interview them, to my mastermind groups for their support, my life and business teachers/mentors T Harv Eker, Loral Langemeier, Jay Abraham, Chet Holmes, Spike Humer, Will Mattox, Joel and Heidi Roberts, Libbe HaLevy, Teri Hawkins, Eric Lofholm, John Carlton, Stan Dahl, and Richard Villasana, Publishing Manager.

PART I

AVOIDING
A CESAREAN

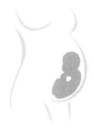

Chapter 1

Cesarean Section: The Real Deal

Congratulations—you're pregnant! This is an exciting time for you, full of the wonder of childbirth…and the anxiety, too. And why shouldn't you feel anxious? You're experiencing major changes to your body, your sleeping habits … pretty much your entire life. You're also being faced with big questions, such as: Are you going to deliver naturally or by cesarean section?

If you're thinking about having a C-section, you're not alone. The procedure is rising in popularity, with an increasing number of women choosing C-sections over vaginal delivery. The U.S. rate has increased by more than half over the last decade; the national average is now 30 percent, and 40 percent in major institutions.[i] Some of my colleagues work at hospitals where the cesarean rate is approaching 50 percent. That means that half of the women who give birth are delivering by C-section!

Unfortunately, this spike in popularity has not been accompanied by better outcomes for mothers *or* babies. In fact the opposite is true. More moms are having more bleeding, recovery is longer, and there's no known benefit to the baby. The USA has one of the worst infant mortality rates of industrialized countries, and the rate for African-Americans is nearly double that of Caucasian women.[ii] The maternal death rate is four times the goal set in 2010 by the U.S. Government's

Healthy People promotion, and far worse—28 to 50 percent of these deaths are preventable.[iii]

As more and more women are having cesarean sections, repeat cesarean sections, and repeat-repeat cesarean sections, their fear and consternation grow with each subsequent procedure. They're faced with the prospect of bleeding, placenta accreta (a severe complication involving an abnormally deep attachment of the placenta), and hysterectomies. With bigger surgeries come longer recovery times, more complications, and problems like infections and chronic pain. For many women, it's an ongoing nightmare, and they've got nowhere to turn.

As a practicing MD and Obstetric Anesthesiologist for more than twenty years, I have personally helped over 24,000 women give birth and been Chief of OB Anesthesia for 100,000 deliveries. I've overseen thousands of C-sections, some more successful than others. The overriding truth is that the better prepared you are, the better outcome you will experience. The more you know, the more prepared and less afraid you'll be. And the less fear you have, the better your birthing experience, whether it's vaginal or cesarean.

That's why I wrote this book: to help you help your baby and yourself. My patients say that I quiet the fears of pregnancy.

I authored *The Safe Baby System* to guide expectant mothers through the complicated process of pregnancy and delivery. In this book, I want to focus on the C-section—what's true, what isn't, and what you need to know. Armed with this knowledge, you'll be better equipped to ask the right questions of your doctor, nurse, or midwife. You'll also be empowered to participate and help improve the safety, control, and quality of your own delivery.

* * *

In my years as an OB Anesthesiologist, I've seen thousands of successful cesarean sections. I have also, unfortunately, seen some that were not successful, and where the outcome could have been avoided with the right preparation. I want to share the following two stories with you.

A few years ago, a young woman named "Anne" wanted to have her second child by VBAC—vaginal birth after cesarean (also now called TOLAC—trial of labor after cesarean). She decided to give birth in a small hospital in New England. Her doctor sent her in to the hospital for induction, but she didn't dilate. So he sent her home.

A couple of days later, he brought her back and tried the induction again, re-starting oxytocin (the same chemical that your body produces naturally during contractions). But this time, Anne's uterus ruptured. The OB was not in the hospital at the time, and because the hospital was not required to, there were no 'house doctors' who could step in as backup. So Anne was forced to wait.

The OB arrived in 30 minutes, but by that point, it was already too late. The baby suffered from hypoxic ischemic encephalopathy, or brain damage.

Stories like Anne's just make you want to cry. But the good news is: it doesn't have to be this way. You can help to ensure that you have a good outcome for you and your baby by knowing the right questions to ask and following the steps laid out in this book. Of course, this book is for education only, and not medical advice. You need to discuss medical questions, treatments and decisions with your personal physician, Obstetrician, or midwife and before beginning any diet, exercise regimen, dietary supplements, or medications.

In Anne's case, tragedy could have been avoided by choosing a different hospital with a better support system. In a larger hospital with dedicated OB Anesthesiologists, labor nurses, scrub techs, and backup doctors available 24/7—either residents in training or "hospitalists" (a new trend)—an obstetric emergency gets handled FAST. That means you can relax, knowing that if a situation develops, you and your baby are in good hands. With the right preparation, the odds are on *your* side.

Take the following story. "Lynette," a doctor's wife, was delivering her firstborn. She was in great shape—she was 5'2" and weighed 130 pounds. Lynette ate well and exercised regularly, and kept herself very active throughout her pregnancy. She decided that vaginal delivery wasn't something she was interested in, so she and her husband scheduled a C-section.

Lynette had the foresight to discuss her pain medications with the OB and hospital staff well before the procedure. She received the medications she wanted during the cesarean, and she continued them into the post-partum period. Facing no complications, she went home on the fourth day with her newborn and only had relatively minor pains.

Within a month or two, Lynette was back into her regular routine and feeling great. She had such a great experience that she had her next two children by cesarean as well. With the right preparation and attitude, a C-section can be a wonderful thing.

* * *

Your doctor, your nurses, and the other hospital staff are all trying very hard to do the best for you. However, human beings are fallible, and the medical system sometimes fails.

It's no one person's fault. Instead, it's a mix of conflicting factors. The trend toward lower reimbursements, increased patient visits, and regulatory pressures to document, document, document add to the stress and hassle of modern medicine. And the big elephant in the room— the threat of a malpractice suit—hangs ever-present in the air.

Nowhere is this truer than in obstetrics. Interestingly, the threat of malpractice suits and the rate of cesarean sections are more closely connected than you might think. A recent study showed that increased malpractice insurance premiums were significantly associated with an increased cesarean rate. In other words, malpractice pressure leads to more cesarean sections.[iv]

Knowing the inside scoop puts you in a far better position to work together with your doctors, midwives, nurses, and others taking care of you. The boat moves forward a lot easier when everyone is paddling in the same direction!

In this book, I want to educate you on all the things to look for—warning signs and the problems you could potentially face. For example, if you know the signs and symptoms of post-partum hemorrhage (bleeding after delivery), then you can help alert the nursing staff and your doctors at the earliest sign of trouble.

C-Section is divided into three parts: Avoiding, Prepare for, and Recovering from a Cesarean. In Part I, I'll give you tips, tools, and strategies for avoiding a cesarean if you hope to have a vaginal birth. Part II is for mothers who choose to have an elective cesarean, as well as those who have a medical indication for one; we'll go over the surgical procedure in detail so that nothing comes as a surprise. **Even if you are planning on having a vaginal birth, you should read this section.** Many women wind up with an unscheduled cesarean, and the better prepared you are, the calmer and more likely you will be able to actively participate. In Part III, we'll focus on how to recover from your C-section so that you and your baby are in great shape. I'll also share certain "Insider Secrets" with you throughout the book—little jewels of wisdom and nuggets of insight that I've gleaned from twenty years of experience.

In these pages, you will learn the steps to take to make sure you are not just another statistic. Through education, empowerment, and asking the right questions, you'll know how to make the right choices. You can reduce your fear and have a great delivery—whether you choose to have your baby naturally or with a cesarean delivery. Your health and the health of your baby are ultimately in your hands.

The more you understand the medical system, the better you can ensure that it serves you, the patient. The more you know, the less stress you have. And the less stress you have, the better the outcome for you and your baby.

Did you know that maternal stress leads to changes in the hormones you release, changing blood flow to the uterus and baby, which in turn can lead to a fetal response to stress and result in poor fetal growth or preterm birth?[vi] Some research even suggests that it can lead to behavioral problems in childhood and as an adult.[vi] But don't panic! Studies also show that you can reduce maternal stress and help have a healthy baby.[vii]

The moral of the story? The more you learn, the less stressed you will be. You will learn to *Quiet the fears of pregnancy*. Not only will you improve your own experience; your baby will thank you as well.

Of course it's normal to be worried. You and your partner are sure to have a million questions spinning through your heads right now. Is the baby going to be okay? Are you? I don't mean to imply that your pregnancy is ever going to be 100 percent stress free. I simply want to minimize those fears and anxieties as much as possible by empowering you. The more active you are in your own care, the more you'll be able to conquer those worries and put them to rest.

That's my goal in *C-Section*: to quiet the fears of pregnancy. The tips and tools you learn in this book will help you keep stress, anxiety, and depression at bay, and help to have a healthy baby.[viii] I want you to be able to enjoy your pregnancy and the birth of your child, no matter what manner of delivery you choose. Whatever your individual fears, I want to help you quiet them; I want to calm the whispers in the back of your mind. Let those nagging thoughts dissipate into the breeze as you bring a new life into the world.

Congratulations—you've taken the first steps toward being a healthy mom, having a healthy baby, and ensuring an easy recovery. To your health!

Now let the journey begin.

Things to Keep In Mind:

- Cesarean sections are increasingly common and can be successful and safe…especially if you are prepared.

- This book will quiet your fears about cesarean sections, so that you'll know what to expect and help to maximize the likelihood of a safe birth.

- The more you know, the more prepared and less afraid you'll be. And the less fear you have, the better your birthing experience, whether it's vaginal or cesarean.

- Fear and Stress is not only not good for you, but also the baby; reducing Fear and Stress will help the baby.

- The book is divided into three sections: Avoiding, Prepare for, and Recover From Cesarean sections.

Go to www.SafeBabySystem.com/bonus for additional information.

REFERENCES

[i] MacDorman MF. Clin Perinatol 2008:35:293-307. Cesarean birth in the United States: epidemiology, trends, and outcomes.

[ii] National Vital Statistics Reports (Nov 24) 2004:53(10):1-8; www.cia.gov/ library/publications/the-world-factbook/rankorder/2091rank.html

[iii] Sentinel Event Alert: 2010:Jan 26th:Issue 44. Preventing Maternal Death. The Joint Commission.

[iv] Yant YT. Med Care. 2009:47:234-42. Relationship between malpractice litigation pressure and rates of Cesarean section and vaginal birth after Cesarean section.

[v] Hobel CJ. Psychosocial Stress and pregnancy outcome. Clin Obstet Gynecol 2008:51:333-348.

[vi] O'Donnell K et al. Prenatal stress and neurodevelopment of the child: focus on the HPA axis and role of the placenta. Dev Neurosci 2009:31:285-292.

[vii] Duncan LG. Mindfulness-based childbirth and parenting education: promoting family mindfulness during the perinatal period. J Child Fam Stud 2010:19:190-202. And O'Donnell K et al. Prenatal stress and neurodevelopment of the child: focus on the HPA axis and role of the placenta. Dev Neurosci 2009:31:285-292.

[viii] Duncan LG. Mindfulness-based childbirth and parenting education: promoting family mindfulness during the perinatal period. J Child Fam Stud 2010:19:190-202. And O'Donnell K et al. Prenatal stress and neurodevelopment of the child: focus on the HPA axis and role of the placenta. Dev Neurosci 2009:31:285-292.

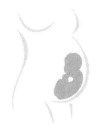

Chapter 2

During Pregnancy: Time to Be Picky

In our discussion of cesarean sections, we're going to start at the beginning. Or, rather, before the beginning has even begun.

If you've already decided that a C-section is how you want to delivery your baby, you may want to skip ahead to Part II of the book. However, I would encourage you to keep reading, just to familiarize yourself with all the options available to you. And if you'd rather not have a cesarean delivery except as a measure of last resort, read on.

Avoiding a cesarean starts long before entering the hospital. It's all about choices—the choices you, the patient, make, and choices made by the team of professionals serving you. This is the part where you're allowed to be picky. And it starts as early as conception. The choices you make before you conceive can dramatically affect your chance of having a cesarean. It all begins . . . by picking the right mate.

Well, okay. By the time you pick up this book, "mate-picking" advice is probably coming a little too late. Nor am I advocating that you pick your mate on the basis of your chances for having a C-section! But it's a simple fact of nature that size does matter. And no, not *that*. I'm talking about that tall, handsome man who desperately wants you to bear his children . . . and whose height won't make it easy to do so.

Think about the basic physics of having a baby through a vaginal delivery. The baby has to fit through the mom's pelvis in the correct orientation and manner, with the head ducking under mom's pubic bone, to get out via the vaginal canal. Giving birth is tougher than a decathlon!

If a 5'2" woman is having a baby with a 6'2" man, the chances are much greater that the baby will be physically tall or large. Thus the baby may not be able to *fit* through the woman's pelvis. We all know that you can't fit a square peg through a round hole; it also deserves to be noted that you can't fit a large object through a small one. Just something to think about if you're still shopping for a mate.

If you've already picked your baby daddy, don't worry: there are still plenty of preemptive measures you can take to make your delivery easier. Remember Lynette from Chapter 1? Even though she chose to have a cesarean, the fact that she was in great shape didn't hurt. And being in good physical shape is even more important if you opt for vaginal delivery.

I'm not kidding when I compare delivery to a decathlon. Labor should be thought of as a physical sport. Could you run a marathon without training? Maybe, but you would probably be beat up, sore, exhausted, and far more prone to injury. The same applies for delivering your baby. The better physical shape you can get into before or even during pregnancy, the better.

You don't have to play extreme sports or start rock-climbing every day. Just choose something that gives you a little aerobic capacity, and that helps build flexibility and strength, especially of your core abdominal muscles (e.g. transverse abdominal muscles) and pelvic floor. This will vastly improve your ability to push, as well as help you avoid injury during pushing (e.g. urinary incontinence, or leakage) and improve your recovery period. A recent study showed that daily pelvic floor exercises done prior to delivery will reduce your chance of urinary incontinence by 40 percent.[i]

Start strengthening your abdominal core and pelvic floor as soon as possible. There are many different paths you can take, such as yoga, Pilates, working with a personal trainer, and exercising with kettlebells.

Make sure your trainer or teacher has additional education about pregnancy exercises. You don't want to be focusing on your 'abs', the rectus abdominus (aka six pack muscles), which some doctors feel can increase your chance for separating those muscles, called rectus diastasis. The core muscles are really about the deeper muscles—the transversus abdominis and the pelvic floor. Kegel exercises are also helpful; these exercises consist of contracting and relaxing the muscles that form part of the pelvic floor. Using these muscles properly will greatly improve your pushing effectiveness, reducing the wear and tear on your body. Many OBs and doctors don't appreciate how the pelvic floor is part of the core muscle group, and the vital importance of training them to strengthen as well as relax. Think about a baby learning to walk—you can't just exercise your thigh and calf muscles, without learning the coordinated motions you need. Knowing the right core exercises can help you to stand better while pregnant, reduce back pain, improve your ability to turn the baby during labor and push, as well as recover faster from vaginal or cesarean birth, with less chance for urinary incontinence later. For an easy, fast, non-impact training program to develop your pelvic floor and core muscles—see the video at www.SafeBabySystem.com/exercises.

This brings me to the subject of pushing. Most women take some sort of class about pregnancy and childbirth. While many of the classes touch upon how to push during labor, they often don't spend enough time on teaching women to push well. Would you expect yourself to have completely mastered basketball or cross-country skiing after one or two short sessions? Probably not.

A great labor coach can make a big difference between successful vaginal delivery and an unplanned trip to the operating room. Studies have shown that continuous labor support can even decrease your chance of having a cesarean.[ii] Your labor coach will help you push, keep you on track, take good care of double-checking your physical comforts

. . . and even give you a massage! Massaging your feet and legs will increase your circulation and help the white blood cells on their journey back to your heart. Aromatherapy, essential oils that smell fantastic, can also be beneficial to your mood.

Regardless of whether you decide to find a professional labor coach or go with the nurse the hospital provides, do yourself (and your baby) a favor and take a class beforehand. Many couples attend Lamaze or Bradley classes. Try to find one that gives more than a cursory review of pushing and breathing. You can also check out the website for more info at www.SafeBabySystem.com.

Eating for Two

Now let's talk about nutrition. One of the best ways to ensure a healthy pregnancy—and to increase your chances for delivering your baby naturally, without invasive surgery—is to watch what you put into your body.

It's the 21st century and everyone knows we should be eating well. But how many of us really do? It's never too late to start eating well. And the sooner you begin, the better off you are. The human body is uniquely wonderful, capable of so much. But like a high-performance car or professional athlete, you have to put quality materials into it. That means organic foods, good quality water, and adequate vitamins and minerals.

A lot of people consume foods that are nutrient deficient, have a high glycemic (sugar) index, and are mineral deficient. It's not your fault. If you go to your supermarket today, the available foods just don't have the same nutritional value as they did in the past. The SAD diet (standard American diet) is rich in sugars, simple carbohydrates, and "bad fats." No wonder the health of the nation has been declining and the obesity rate has skyrocketed in recent years.

It's a myth (albeit a popular myth) that when you're pregnant, you can eat whatever you want. Yes, you may be craving two buckets of ice cream, but now it's more important than ever that you eat the right foods. After all, you're eating for two.

What you want to consume is more of the "good fats," like the omega-3s found in fish oil. "What?" you say. "I don't want ANY fats in my body. I'm pregnant—I already feel fat enough!"

But the good fats are on *your* side. They're the basic building blocks of staying fit and healthy. Your body processes these building blocks into more complex molecules that control innumerable functions throughout the body. An overabundance of bad fats leads to inflammatory processes, diseases, and can even contribute to premature labor. The good fats, on the other hand, found in fish oil, flax seed, walnuts, salmon, mackerel, sardines, walnut oil, canola oil and even smaller amounts in soybeans, Tofu, spinach and kale,[iii] are used by the body to make anti-inflammatory compounds.

Studies have proven that good fats bring with them a variety of good effects. DHA (an omega-3 fatty acid) is particularly beneficial. DHA and other good fats are used to make fetal brain and eye tissue, and they've even been linked to longer pregnancies.[iv] Don't just increase your good fats, remember to cut down on the bad fats too. Your body responds to the ratio of good fat to bad fat, altering their metabolism, changing the downstream chemical building blocks that can help you and your baby be healthy and happy.

But enough about fat. Now let's talk about sugar. A food's average sugar load is called the glycemic index. Foods like ice cream and sugary cereals are not only high in calories; they also have a high glycemic index, meaning that the body absorbs the sugar quickly, leading to an increased blood sugar level. The glycemic index of the food you eat has a lot to do with gaining or losing weight and the development of diabetes and heart disease. It can even increase pregnancy problems such as macrosomia (big baby), preeclampsia (high blood pressure during pregnancy), and, of course, cesarean section.

The glycemic index of foods is a great way to manage and make wise choices about what you eat. For instance, a plain potato is composed of simple starches. These taste good, but they're easily absorbed. After you eat that tasty potato, it may be out of mind, but it's definitely not out of your system. Your blood sugar increases, and you pump more insulin to tell your body's cells to take up the sugar out of the blood and store in—not only as glycogen in the liver, but also as fat!

Over time, you can "burn out" your ability to release enough insulin to maintain a normal blood sugar. This happens because your body develops an "insulin resistance"—it takes a higher and higher amount of insulin to normalize your blood sugar. In the early years, they called this Syndrome X, later to be renamed Metabolic Syndrome. Today this has been well-documented as the inevitable outcome of years of eating poorly, and often the path to diabetes, heart disease, and death.

There are pregnancy-specific risks, too. Running a high glucose during very early pregnancy can lead to increased fetal loss and a greater chance of congenital malformations. The elevated blood sugar alters the key proteins in your baby, which can negatively affect the embryology and development of the fetus in the first six to ten weeks. Diabetes during pregnancy also tends to lead to large babies, which increased your chances for a cesarean.

And all that from a potato!

In contrast, a sweet potato has a low glycemic index. That means the carbohydrates are absorbed more slowly, resulting in a lower blood sugar level for you. So by substituting yams for baked potatoes, you'll be making a smart choice for you and your baby.

It's important to learn more about the glycemic index of the foods you eat during your pregnancy. A good source of information is the "Get the Healthy Edge" program created by Amber Thiel, available at www.GetTheHealthyEdge.com. The Healthy Edge vision is about reversing the national obesity trend by encouraging Americans to take responsibility for their health.

It's not an exaggeration to say that obesity is an American epidemic. An estimated 34 percent of Americans are obese, with over 5 percent being morbidly obese.[v] And obesity is no friend to the pregnant mother—it can result in complications, cesarean section, and even the death of your baby. If obesity is something you struggle with, commit yourself to doing what it takes to get down to a reasonable weight. Another great friend and resource are Annette Sym's cookbooks at www.symplytoogood.com. Even if it is too late to lose weight, not easy under any circumstance, the steps in *The Safe Baby System* will still guide you to help ensure not only a healthy baby, but also that you're around for a long time to watch your children grow up and have babies of their own!

Checking In for a Check-Up

Now that you're exercising and eating right, you're well on the way to having a problem-free, natural delivery. Next on your To Do list is to familiarize yourself with your medical history and make sure everything is up to snuff.

More and more pregnant women today have preexisting medical conditions. The prevalence of preexisting medical conditions in women giving birth has increased 20 percent, affecting almost 200,000 women a year in the USA.[vi] If this describes you, it isn't a bad thing. It just means you have a little more prep work to do to make sure everything goes off without a hitch.

If you have medical diseases such as diabetes, heart disease, or kidney disease, it's best to get them tuned up and optimized as soon as possible. Ideally, this should happen before you get pregnant, but the sooner the better.

If you have significant medical problems, be sure to schedule a consultation with your anesthesiologist well before you could go into labor. Additional tests may be needed or certain medications changes before your due date. During this consultation, you can discuss your specific medical problems and the choices available to you, which will alleviate many of your fears.

Women with preexisting medical conditions often have significantly more fear during their pregnancies than women who don't. Fear is the enemy of the pregnant mother. It's not just an annoyance; it's a health hazard. Because fear causes an increase in stress hormones, it also causes an increase in glucocorticoid hormones, which increases your blood sugar—and we've already discussed the dangers associated with high blood sugar during pregnancy. Hormones like cortisol have been shown to cross the placenta and may cause long-term development changes, increasing your child's risk of attention deficit disorder/hyperactivity, anxiety, and language delay.[vii]

To make matters worse, stress hormones like adrenalin and noradrenalin can actually decrease blood flow to the uterus and baby. New scientific information linking the physiologic responses of maternal stress to premature births have shown that stress can increase the chances of premature birth by 50 to 100 percent![viii]

Then there's preeclampsia, one of the biggest risks today's pregnant mothers face. Preeclampsia is a hypertensive (high blood pressure) disorder of pregnancy, which can be worsened by stress, diabetes, and other preexisting medical problems. Statistically, it is the second highest-ranking cause of death to pregnant women. Severe preeclampsia has increased nearly 50 percent, affecting over 36,000 women annually in the USA.[ix]

I want to share with you the tragic story of "Beth," a woman with twins—which is one of the risk factors for preeclampsia. Late in her last trimester, Beth came in to the hospital for nausea and vomiting. She had some blood work done, an ultrasound, and a non-stress test, and everything checked out—her blood pressure was normal. So she was sent home.

However, two days later Beth was back with the same symptoms. When they checked her into the hospital and looked in the computer, they saw that the blood work done two days earlier was abnormal. Her liver enzymes were elevated, indicating HELLP syndrome (Hemolysis, Elevated Liver enzymes, and Low Platelets), a severe form of preeclampsia. They drew her blood again, and her OB took her immediately to the operating room (OR) for a cesarean.

The twins were born without difficulty: two perfectly healthy baby boys. Unfortunately, because no one followed up the labs the first time, her liver had gotten very damaged over the previous two days. She went into liver failure and, after a heroic battle in the ICU, passed away.

Beth's death is a warning sign to all of us. Humans make tragic mistakes every day, and the humans in hospitals are no different. That's why it's imperative that you know exactly what tests are being done to you.

> ### INSIDER SECRET
>
> Don't let the statistics scare you. In spite of dangers like preeclampsia, the vast majority of expectant mothers are just fine after delivering their babies. In 2006, the U.S. Department of Health and Human Services reported that the maternal mortality rate was 13.3 out of 100,000 live births. That's 0.013 percent or 1 in 7500.

Write down the names and ask for the results. You may not need to know the exact numbers, but if a doctor or midwife or even your primary care provider thinks a test is important enough to order, you deserve to know that the result was followed, checked, and that each test was normal. If it wasn't normal, you deserve to be told the medical plan that will be followed next.

It's important to be aware of the signs of preeclampsia so that you can notify your doctor right away. Once in the hospital, you will be monitored closely, but in the months leading up to your delivery, you are your own monitor between prenatal visits. Warning signs include high blood pressure, protein in urine, sudden weight gain (water weight), severe swelling of the legs or face, hyperreflexia (e.g. exaggerated knee jerk reflex), headaches, nausea, blurry vision/seeing spots, or pain in your upper abdomen. Your doctor or midwife will be checking for protein in the urine with a simple dip stick test on office visits or send it out to the lab. If you feel you have any signs of preeclampsia, call your doctor or midwife right away.

The origins of preeclampsia start very early in pregnancy—probably when the placenta abnormally implants into the uterus. Later, the body develops a reaction against the placenta, resulting in constriction of the blood vessels and high blood pressure. Some studies have shown that oxidative stress is a key component of preeclampsia, and that antioxidants taken early in pregnancy may help prevent the onset of the disorder.[x]

If you've been unable to stem severe preeclampsia during your pregnancy the condition may warrant a cesarean section. Indications of severe preeclampsia include:

- very high blood pressure (>160/110 mmHg),

- high protein in the urine (>3-5 grams/24-hour urine, or 3-4+ on urine dipstick),

- worsening clinical symptoms of pain around the stomach,

- worsening severity of headaches,

- seeing spots (visual changes).

Certain blood tests may be abnormal as well, such as the liver enzymes (as was the case for Beth), platelet count, or red blood cell count. These are all common signs of HELLP. And if you're experiencing them, get help ASAP!

Does preeclampsia automatically mean you'll need a cesarean? Not at all. But if your delivery is not moving along the way your doctor would like it to, you may require one. Preeclampsia is nothing to fool around with. Stress makes preeclampsia worse.

Often the antidote is surprisingly simple: educate and prepare yourself. If you have a preexisting medical condition, approaching your fears head-on is the best way to overcome them. The better prepared you are, the less stressed you will be. And the best place to start is by having an in-depth conversation with your OB or midwife about how to ensure the best possible outcome for you and your baby. Which brings us to our next topic in our discussion of how to avoid a cesarean: finding the perfect doctor or midwife to usher your baby into the world.

Vetting the Hired Help

We've talked about selecting the right partner in terms of the father of your child. Now let's talk about selecting another kind of partner: the kind with the credentials.

One of the most important factors that will determine whether you wind up having a vaginal or a cesarean delivery is who your obstetrician or midwife is—all the more reason to choose well.

Different obstetricians have different experiences and thresholds for what they will let you or the baby tolerate before pushing the cesarean section decision button. We are all influenced by our experiences, as well as what the modern literature says. Some OBs are more comfortable with assisted deliveries (e.g., forceps or vacuum) than others.

When my wife was pregnant for the first time, we picked our OB for not only being a nice guy and all-around excellent physician, but also for his ability to use forceps. And of course, wouldn't you know it: he needed to use forceps during the delivery of our first child, a whopping 8.6-pound baby girl. Another OB may have chosen to do a cesarean, which, in our particular case, would have caused greater trauma to my wife and daughter.

Skill in forceps was a priority for me and my wife. You'll have your own list of priorities. One thing you'll want to be sure to talk to your OB about is their policies on induction of labor, another biggie. Over 22 percent of women have labor induced.[xi] The reasons vary—sometimes there are definitive medical indications for induction of labor, but this is not always the case. A reasonable rule of thumb —induction is indicated when the prolongation of the pregnancy is not healthy for mom or baby and there are no contraindications to induction.[xii] See Figure 2.1 for more details.[xiii]

INDICATIONS FOR INDUCTION	DRUGS FOR INDUCTION
Placental abruption, mild (partial separation of placenta from uterus)	**Cervical Ripening:** *Mechanical* **laminaria (sponge that slowly swells up), Foley balloon in cervix**
Chorioamnionitis (infection in placenta and membranes)	
High blood pressure of pregnancy (gestational, preeclampsia, eclampsia)	*Chemical* **Misoprostol 25 mcg– NOT TO BE USED IF PRIOR CESAREAN!!!**
Post-term pregnancy >41 weeks	**Dinoprostone**
Maternal medical conditions (e.g. diabetes)	**Oxytocin starting dose: low dose 2 mU/min high dose 6 mU/min, may**
Fetal compromise (not doing as well as he/she should be; e.g. IUGR growth restriction, Oliogohydram-nios—low amniotic fluid)	**increase >every 15 minutes. Local practices vary.**
Logistical reasons (Convenience)—but not before 39 weeks without proof of fetal lung maturity	
Note: not an all inclusive list. Consult with your OB or midwife.	

Figure 2. 1

There is an increasing use of induction of labor for convenience—Dad is going out of town, Grandma is coming into town, Mom is tired of being pregnant, or the OB's working under a tight schedule. While both technique and reliability have improved the success rate of inductions that successfully result in a vaginal delivery, it may not be the same as natural labor. Be sure to discuss this thoroughly with your OB.

Years ago, when I was working in New York, inductions used to be a three-day process. We'd turn on the Pitocin (oxytocin) all day, turn it off at night, turn it back on the next day, turn if off that night, and by the third day, the mother either delivered vaginally or we'd do a cesarean. The reason we'd turn the oxytocin off at night is to reduce the chance for uterine atony. With uterine atony, the uterus does not respond to contraction medications like oxytocin, causing the mom to bleed after delivery and sometimes requiring a blood transfusion or even a hysterectomy . . . all because labor had been induced.

Fortunately, the technique has improved. Today, there are agents to help "ripen" the cervix. Prostaglandins like cervadil and misoprostil can be placed in the vagina to help soften the cervix. Success rates for induction of labor are much higher when the cervix is considered favorable or "ripe", especially with a favorable Bishop Score (rating of cervix).[xiv]

> **INSIDER SECRET**
>
> If you are planning an elective Cesarean, be sure you are at least at 39 weeks gestation. Some C-sections are scheduled as early as 38 or even 37 weeks, but the data overwhelming shows that it is better for the baby to wait until 39 weeks. A recent article showed increased risk to the baby for neonatal death, respiratory complication, low blood sugar, infection and admission to the Neonatal Intensive Care Unit (NICU) at 37 weeks (double the risk) or even at 38 weeks (risk increased by 50 percent) compared to 39 weeks gestation.
>
> Tita A. Timing of Elective Repeat Cesarean Delivery at Term and Neonatal Outcomes. NEJM 2009:360:111-20.

So let's lay out the three basic questions you'll want to ask your OB. These are the questions you'll first discuss with your partner, and then with the "partner" in the white coat. When you're choosing who is going to deliver your baby, ask them:

- What is your cesarean section rate?
- How many deliveries do you do a year?
- Who covers you if you are away, and what is their cesarean section rate?

INSIDER SECRET

There are certain preemptive measures you can take to decrease your chances for premature labor. Start taking a daily supplement of fish oil. Next, find ways to reduce your stress level, whether through yoga, meditation, or taking long walks. Also, be alert to signs of vaginal infections (which can spread to uterus and induce premature labor). One way to ward off infection is to take good bacteria (probiotics) that can help colonize your intestines, colon, and vaginal canal with the good guys, reducing the risk for vaginal and endometrial infection.

Saling E. The Lactobacilli-Protection system of pregnant women – efficient prevention of premature births by early detection of disturbances. Z Geburtsh Neonataol 2005:209:128-34. and Leitich H, Bacterial vaginosis as a risk factor for pre- term delivery: a meta-analysis. Am J Obstet Gynecol 2003:189:139-47. And Trenev N. Probiotics: nature's internal healers. Avery Publishing Group. Garden City Park, NY 1998.

Most OBs will do a cesarean section if you are going to deliver prematurely and the baby is in the breech position (butt down instead of head down). While the baby is still small and able to flip around, breech position is pretty common. If your baby is in breech and you go into labor, there isn't much you can do, although some acupuncturists claim good success at turning a breech baby into proper position before labor begins.

It's important that you and your OB discuss the indications for a cesarean. Breech position is just one of many; others include macrosomia (large baby), multiple gestation (twins or more), prior cesareans, placenta previa (placenta covers internal opening of cervix, so the baby has no way out), and more (see Figure 2.2).[xv] Again, a good rule of thumb: a cesarean is indicated when delivery must be accomplished (for baby or mom reasons) and the risks of induction or additional labor are greater than the risk of a cesarean.[xvi] Each OB will have a different level of tolerance. What are the indications for *your* doctor? What are the emergency scenarios in which she will order a C-section pronto?

Indications for Cesarean Delivery

Fetal Reasons
Not tolerating labor—"non reassuring fetal status",
Category III tracing
Prolapsed umbilical cord
Breech or transverse position of baby (not head down)
Risk of fetal infection (mom has active genital herpes, HIV not well-controlled)
Congenital anomalies that would make passing through birth canal difficult or dangerous
Failed Vacuum or Forceps
Failure to progress (cervical dilatation, or descent with pushing)

Maternal-Fetal Reasons
Mechanical obstruction to vaginal delivery (e.g. Fibroid, Large baby, CPD)
CPD (celphalo-pelvic distortion)—baby won't fit through mom's pelvis
Placenta problems—separation (abruption); blocking cervix (previa)
Bleeding
Uterine Rupture

Maternal Reasons
To protect mom's health (rare—e.g., brain tumor, severe heart disease)
Elective (maternal request)
Repeat Cesarean
Previous Uterine surgery/scar not in a low transverse position
Note: not an all inclusive list. Consult with your OB or midwife.

Figure 2. 2

INSIDER SECRET

Is there a certain time of day when Cesareans are more prevalent? Sure—when daily life comes into play. There tend to be more requests for C-sections before midnight, after dinner, and before office hours. Many OBs prefer to do Cesareans before or after office hours, not in the middle of the office day. Have you ever had to wait longer or have your appointment cancelled because your doctor was stuck in surgery? Now you know why.

Then, of course, there are the C-sections for which there is no medical indication.[xxvii] Over 6 percent of women choose to have a C-section out of fear of possible problems during labor and vaginal delivery—like a stretched or torn vagina and rectum or urinary incontinence later in life. Other women do so because it's more convenient. Our lives are so busy and complex that sometimes the ability to control one not-so-minor event is a blessing. Just make an appointment, go in, and have the baby. The in-laws can nab a great deal on airline tickets, everyone is there at exactly the right time, and your baby comes on *your* timetable.

In this section we're focusing our attention on avoiding C-sections, but let me say a quick word to mothers who are leaning toward having the surgery. The risks and benefits are unique to you, as is the decision. Just be sure to discuss it thoroughly with your OB or midwife and gather all the information you possibly can so that you're as well-informed as can be.

As you hand-pick your birthing team, it's also important that you choose the right place to have your baby. (For further information on choosing between a hospital, a birthing center, and a home delivery, refer to Chapter 6 of *The Safe Baby System.*) If you have previously had a cesarean and are now seeking a natural delivery, you must be particularly vigilant in selecting the right OB and hospital. Many doctors and hospitals have stopped offering VBACs—vaginal birth after cesareans. Most of the larger, well-known hospitals still perform VBACs, but many smaller ones don't. American Congress of Obstetricians and Gynecologists

(ACOG) estimates that 34 percent of hospitals have fewer than 500 deliveries per year, and providing comprehensive care is frequently impossible.[xviii]

After the 2001 ACOG Committee Opinion stated that in order to perform a VBAC, the OB, Anesthesiologist (physician), or CRNA (nurse) needed to be immediately available, many OBs and smaller hospitals stopped offering VBACs.[xix] They just don't have the 24-hour in-hospital staff to provide immediate cesarean in case of an emergency.

The main concern is uterine rupture. Any scar on the uterus—not just ones from a prior cesarean—can put you at risk for uterine rupture when you go into labor. Even a simple myomectomy (excision of uterine fibroid) can leave a scar that can tear. I've heard OBs exclaim countless times what a good choice it was for a woman to have an elective repeat cesarean because, once they began the surgery, they saw that the uterine wall had already thinned into a membranous "window" long before they'd had any contractions. Undoubtedly these moms would have been dealing with a ruptured uterus had they gone into labor, which would have put their baby's life at risk.

How often does uterine rupture actually occur? With a second indicated cesarean—meaning, the mother had wanted to have a VBAC but needed to have a C-section at the last minute—the risk of uterine rupture is 0.12 percent, compared to 0.02 for an elective repeat cesarean. They generally don't allow a VBAC after two cesareans as the rate of rupture rises to 1-3.7 percent.[xxi] The type of previous uterine incision also matters; although the vast majority are lower uterine now, a classical (head to toe) incision increases the uterine rupture rate to 4-9 percent.

If you've had a prior cesarean and plan to have an induction of labor, be especially careful. Uterine rupture was nearly five times higher in women having a VBAC with induction by oxytocin than in women having an elective repeat cesarean. But don't let the statistics scare you: the rate is still less than 1 percent for both groups. Just be aware that certain drugs have certain effects. Agents that help ripen the cervix—prostaglandins—increase the likelihood of rupture to 24.5 out of 1,000: fifteen times higher than a repeat cesarean.[xxii] If you are having a VBAC and the doctor uses Pitocin (oxytocin) to augment or increase the frequency and strength of contractions, the chance for uterine rupture increases by two to three times.

It's important that you know the signs of uterine rupture. Classically, one of the hallmarks of uterine rupture is abdominal pain that is more than usual, especially pain that is persistent and hard to treat. A misshapen uterus, changes in fetal heart rate (e.g., a non-reassuring pattern, especially with bradycardia), and hypotension can all be signs. Uterine ruptures can cause internal blood loss of up to one liter of blood,[xxiv] and a crash cesarean becomes immediately necessary.

The baby is in danger during uterine rupture. Though the risk of outcomes like stillbirth, brain damage, and neonatal death is only 0.27 percent, it should not be taken lightly.[xxv] Uterine rupture is a very serious event—both baby and mom are at risk for severe bleeding and death. Even though the absolute risk is small, the consequences are very grave.

That's why if you choose to have a VBAC, also called a TOLAC (trial of labor after cesarean), it's crucial to make sure the hospital you choose has all the right support people ON the premises 24/7. In the past, national societies and regulatory agencies have allowed some wiggle room as to the definition of "immediately available"; it was generally up to each hospital to decide what that meant.

But it isn't all gloom and doom. The benefits of a successful VBAC are many. They usually mean a faster, easier recovery, with earlier discharge home. Because you are not having surgery, there is generally less bleeding, pain, and immobilization. And once you've have a successful VBAC, the coast is clear for subsequent VBACs, too.

These are all important things to know as you think about your options. The more you know, the calmer you'll be. Remember that when emotion runs high, intellect runs low. By learning the language of cesareans, you'll be calm and in the loop. Remember to keep the lines of communication with your doctor or midwife open so that you know the exact emergency scenarios in which he or she will default to a cesarean delivery. Once again: knowledge is power. Knowing exactly what to ask for—and how much of it—can make the difference between a rough and a smooth delivery. We'll discuss this in more depth in the next chapter.

Things To Keep In Mind

- Avoiding a cesarean begins during early pregnancy. The right exercise program can help you avoid a cesarean later on.

- A great labor coach can make a big difference between successful vaginal delivery and an unplanned trip to the operating room.

- Healthy nutrition, organic foods, good quality water, and adequate vitamins and minerals, makes a big difference.

- Get a full checkup as early as possible in your pregnancy; failing to deal with health issues increases both fear as well as the possibility of complications.

- Choosing the right OB and hospital is vitally important.

- You can have a VBAC under the right circumstances, which will make delivery easier and hasten your recovery.

Go to www.SafeBabySystem.com/bonus for additional information.

REFERENCES

[i] Wilson PD, Herbison RM, Herbison GP. Obstetric practice and the prevalence of urinary incontinence three months after delivery. Br J Obstet Gynaecol. 1996Feb;103(2):154-61.

[ii] McGrath SK. Birth 2008:35:92-97. A randomized controlled trial of continuous labor support for middle-class couples: effect on cesarean delivery rates.

[iii] http://www.tufts.edu/med/nutrition-infection/hiv/health_omega3.html accessed September 1, 2010

[iv] Lucas M, Dewailly E, Muckle G, et al. Gestation age and birth weight in relation to n-=3 fatty acids among Inuit (Canada). Lipids 2004:39:617-26 and Facchinetti F, Fazzio M, Venturini P. Polyunsaturated fatty acids and risk of preterm delivery. Eur Rev Med Pharacol Sci 2005:9:41-8 and Olsen SF, Soorensen JF, Secher NJ, et al. Fish oil supplementation and duration of pregnancy. A randomized controlled trial. Ugeskr Laeger 1994:156:1302.

[v] Flegal KM. Prevalence and trends in obesity among US adults, 1999-2008. *JAMA* 2010;303:235-241.

[vi] Berg CJ. Obstet Gynecol 2009113:1075-81. Overview of maternal morbidity during hospitalization for labor and delivery in the United States 1993-1997 and 2001-2005.

[vii] O'Donnell K et al. Prenatal stress and neurodevelopment of the child: focus on the HPA axis and role of the placenta. Dev Neurosci 2009:31:285-292. And Hobel CJ. Psychosocial Stress and pregnancy outcome. Clin Obstet Gynecol 2008:51:333-348. And Talge NM and the Early Stress, Translational Research and prevention science network: fetal and neonatal experience on child and adolescent mental health. Antenatal maternal stress and long-term effects on child neurodevelopment: how and why? J Child Psychology and Psychiatry. 2007:48:245-61.

[viii] Hobel CJ. Psychosocial Stress and pregnancy outcome. Clin Obstet Gynecol 2008:51:333-348. AND Hobel C. Role of psychosocial and nutritional stress on poor pregnancy outcome. J Nutr 2003:133:1709S-1717S.

[ix] Berg CJ. Obstet Gynecol 2009113:1075-81.

[x] Bodnar LM et al. 2006. Periconceptional multivitamin use reduces the risk of preeclampsia. Am J Epidemiology 164:470–7. And Chappell LC, Seed PT, Kelly FJ et al. 2002. Vitamin C and E supplementation in women at risk of preeclampsia is associated with changes in indices of oxidative stress and placental function. Am J Obstet Gynecol 187:777–84. And Chappell LC, Seed PT, Briley AL et al. 1999. Effect of antioxidants on the occurrence of preeclampsia in women at increased risk: a randomized trial. Lancet 394:810–16.

[xi] ACOG Practice Bulletin, NUMBER 107, AUGUST 2009 Induction of Labor.

[xii] Thorp JM. Chapter 36. Clinical aspects of normal and abnormal labor. In Creasy & Resnik's maternal-fetal medicine: principles and practice 6th Edition. 2009. Saunders Elsevier. Philadelphia. P701.

[xiii] ACOG Committee Opinion Number 342, August 2006 *(Replaces No. 271, April 2002)* Induction of Labor for Vaginal Birth After Cesarean Delivery and ACOG Practice Bulletin, NUMBER 107, AUGUST 2009 Induction of Labor and Battista LR, Wing DA. Chapter 13. Abnormal labor and induction of labor. In Gabbe: Obstetrics normal and problem pregnancies, 5th Edition. Edited by Gabbe S, Niebyl J, Simpson J. Churchill Livingstone Philadelphia 2007, P322-343.

[xiv] ACOG Practice Bulletin, NUMBER 107, AUGUST 2009 Induction of Labor and Battista LR, Wing DA. Chapter 13. Abnormal labor and induction of labor. In Gabbe: Obstetrics normal and problem pregnancies, 5th Edition. Edited by Gabbe S, Niebyl J, Simpson J. Churchill Livingstone Philadelphia 2007, P322-343.

[xv] Landon, M. Chapter 19 Cesarean Delivery. in Gabbe: Obstetrics: normal and problem pregnancies, 5th Ed. Edited by Gabbe S, Niebyl J, Simpson J. Churchill Livingstone Philadelphia 2007, p486-520. and http://en.wikipedia.org/ wiwi/Caesarean_section accessed November 23, 2010.

[xvi] Thorp JM. Chapter 36. Clinical aspects of normal and abnormal labor. In Creasy & Resnik's maternal-fetal medicine: principles and practice 6th Edition. 2009. Saunders Elsevier. Philadelphia.

[xvii] Landon, M. Chapter 19 Cesarean Delivery. in Gabbe: Obstetrics: normal and problem pregnancies, 5th Ed. Edited by Gabbe S, Niebyl J, Simpson J. Churchill Livingstone Philadelphia 2007, p486-520.

[xviii] ACOG Committee Opinion Number 433 • May 2009 • *(Replaces No. 256, May 2001)* Optimal Goals for Anesthesia Care in Obstetrics.

[xix] ACOG Committee Opinion Number 433 • May 2009 • *(Replaces No. 256, May 2001)* Optimal Goals for Anesthesia Care in Obstetrics.

[xx] Spong CY. Risk of uterine rupture and adverse perinatal outcome at term after Cesarean delivery. Obstet Gynecol 2007;110:801-7.

[xxi] ACOG Practice Bulletin. Clinical Management Guidelines For Obstetrician—Gynecologists Number 54, July 2004 *(Replaces Practice Bulletin Number 5, July 1999)* Vaginal Birth After Previous Cesarean Delivery.

[xxii] ACOG Practice Bulletin. Clinical Management Guidelines For Obstetrician—Gynecologists Number 54, July 2004 *(Replaces Practice Bulletin Number 5, July 1999)* Vaginal Birth After Previous Cesarean Delivery.

[xxiii] ACOG Committee Opinion Number 342, August 2006 *(Replaces No. 271, April 2002)* Induction of Labor for Vaginal Birth After Cesarean Delivery.

[xxiv] Francois KE and Foley MR. Chapter 18. Antepartum and Postpartum Hemorrhage in Gabbe: Obstetrics: normal and problem pregnancies, 5th Ed. Edited by Gabbe S, Niebyl J, Simpson J. Churchill Livingstone Philadelphia 2007, p456-487.

[xxv] Spong CY. Risk of uterine rupture and adverse perinatal outcome at term after Cesarean delivery. Obstet Gynecol 2007;110:801-7.

[xxvi] ACOG Committee Opinion Number 433 • May 2009 • *(Replaces No. 256, May 2001)* Optimal Goals for Anesthesia Care in Obstetrics.

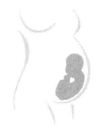

Chapter 3

During Labor: Learn the Lingo

So push has come to shove (no pun intended), and you're in labor. You've decided to bring your son or daughter into the world the natural way. In this chapter, we're going to discuss specific, actionable tools to take with you into the delivery room to ensure that you and your baby stay healthy during labor. I'm going to share with you a number of ways to decrease your chances for an emergency cesarean and clear any obstacles that stand between you and a normal vaginal delivery.

It's All in a Name

Let's start with the basics: vocabulary. Familiarizing yourself with some of the words you might hear in the delivery room will help you stay informed as to what's going on. Not only is this the best way to eliminate ignorance and fear; it also gives you the upper hand when it seems like the hospital staff is "talking around the patient," something that most doctors (and some nurses, too)

INSIDER SECRET

Here's an interesting fact: over 85 percent of women receive continuous fetal monitoring in labor despite no proven benefit to the baby, compared to intermittent checking of the baby's heart rate. (Rev Obstet Gynecol. 2008;1(4): 186-192) Why is it so common? You guessed it—medicolegal concerns! But did you know that continuous monitoring has been shown to increase the Cesarean rate? (Am J Obstet Gynecol 1979:124:399) Definitely something to consider as you go into labor and delivery!

have a tendency to do. By learning some of the terminology and tracing patterns that warrant an emergency cesarean section, as well as those that don't. See www.SafeBabySystem.com for additional information. That way you can discuss with your doctor the need for a cesarean, or whether you and your baby are doing well enough that you can wait a little while until the situation improves.

Some of the terminology has recently changed. The once-prevalent term "fetal distress" is imprecise at best; it has now been replaced by "non-reassuring fetal status," which is accompanied by additional descriptions.[i] Instead of just referring to decels (FHR, or fetal heart rate, deceleration), the patterns are described and then fitted into Categories I, II, or III. These categories describe the urgency of what's going on. Category I means Normal, Category II means Indeterminate, and Category III means Abnormal. Category 1 is normal, with a fetal heart rate 110-160 beats per minute, FHR variability (a good sign), and no bad types of decels, or fetal heart rate drops. Category II does not tell you if things are good or bad. A Category III tracing is abnormal, associated with low fetal pH (acid, meaning baby not doing well). A Category III tracing show no FHR variability (lack of a good sign) and fetal decels that are undesirable (late, variable, or bradycardia – low heart rate). A Category III tracing is an abnormal FHR tracing that requires intervention – starting with intrauterine resuscitation of the fetus (see below). If the baby shows no improvement soon, you need a cesarean or prompt vaginal delivery.[ii]

While you don't have to become an expert in fetal heart rate patterns, it's helpful to be familiar with the terms in case they come up during your labor. That way you can either help the staff avoid a cesarean or help to make having a cesarean happen faster.

"*Intrauterine resuscitation of the fetus*" sounds fancy, but it simply means intervention. If you're at a Category III, then the doctor and nursing team needs to intervene to maximize the oxygen flowing to the baby quickly in order to avoid a cesarean. In terms of fetal distress, there are five things to do.

1. Give oxygen to the baby by giving an oxygen mask to mom;

2. Increase the IV fluids—more fluid to circulate around mom's body to the uterus and placenta;

3. Change of position—by moving the weight of the baby off mom's inferior vena cava (major low pressure venous blood vessel on the right side of the spine) or possibly off an umbilical cord, you can improve blood flow to the baby;

4. Relax the uterus if it is contracted—prolonged or frequent contractions of the uterus decrease the amount of blood flow and oxygen getting to the baby. The uterus can be relaxed by giving terbutaline (0.25 milligrams IV/IM – intra-muscular) or nitroglycerin (100 micrograms) intravenously or by sublingual (beneath the tongue) spray.

5. Raise mom's blood pressure if it's low—the baby is dependent upon the blood flow to the uterus, and it's got to maintain the right pressure. Blood pressure can be increased by giving fluids, but also by giving vasopressors (medication), such as ephedrine and phenylephrine, intravenously.

You don't need an RN or MD degree to be caught up on what's happening in the delivery room. Knowing the basic terms and vocabulary will help you keep up with what's going on and watch for problems. You and your partner will be able to stay on top of things—even if you're under a lot of pressure at the time.

Epidurals: The Enduring Myths

Epidurals, as we all know, can be used to take away the pain of contractions at any point during labor. Much has been written about the correlation between epidurals and cesareans. Let me put these myths to rest: epidurals do not cause C-sections.

Early studies showed that there was in fact an association between epidural use and cesarean sections, but they do not cause them. A woman who has a fast, less painful labor may not need an epidural. Meanwhile, women with slower, more painful labors are way more likely to get an epidural for the pain. And that's where the line between cause and effect begins to blur. Because slow, painful labors—also called dysfunctional labors—are more likely to wind up with a cesarean, whether or not they get an epidural! The primary cause is the type of labor itself; the need for pain relief is a secondary phenomenon.

The higher-quality studies have clearly shown that epidurals *do not cause* cesarean sections. Indeed, even ACOG states definitely that "more recent studies have shown that epidural analgesia does not increase the risks of cesarean delivery."[iii] Many doctors, nurses and midwives even say that an epidural can help you dilate your cervix by letting you relax during labor, instead of fighting the pain.

That said, there are certain problem signs that you should be aware of, and minor things that you can help with. For example, your blood pressure needs to be checked before, during, and after an epidural. The epidural causes vasodilation of your blood vessels. That's why you need to get 500-1000 ml of fluid intravenously before your epidural. It's key to maintain a normal blood pressure. The fluid essentially allows you to "fill up the tank" of the dilated blood vessels in order to maintain the return of blood to the heart, and ultimately through the body to the uterus.

Of course a perplexing problem can be: what is your "normal" blood pressure? Oftentimes when you are in pain (like right before getting an epidural), your blood pressure is elevated because of the pain. So pay attention to what your blood pressure has been running in the office on your prenatal visits, and what it was in early labor. That way you can make sure your blood pressure stays close to normal in order to maximize blood flow to the uterus and baby. While many doctors will tell you anything above 100 mmHg systolic (top number of 100/60) is fine, you really want it to be within 15 percent of your normal blood pressure.

Sometimes your breathing can feel weird after an epidural. Usually that's caused by some amount of numbing medicine affecting the sensation of your chest wall moving. On very rare occasions, this may be a red flag of a high-level or spinal effect of the epidural, which could be dangerous if left unattended. It's best to play it safe. If your breathing feels unusual or labored, let your nurse or anesthesiologist know. For more information about pain relief options see *The Safe Baby System Chapter 12: Pain Relief from A to Z.*

Your Dynamic Duo

Unless you've chosen to have a home delivery, there are probably going to be a lot of faces in the delivery room. Because these people will all be doing their part to ensure a safe, natural delivery, it's helpful to familiarize yourself with a couple of the key players.

Your nurse in labor is your best ally and your first line of defense. She is responsible for taking care of you on many levels—she's looking out for your interest, as well as your baby's, and she's helping the doctors, too. Having a great nurse can make all the difference in the delivery room. And if you talk to your nurse beforehand and let them know that you're trying to avoid a cesarean, she'll do everything in her power to keep you on course.

Some nurses have special "tricks" to help position you so the baby will turn, or to help the baby "drop down." Other nurses have tricks for helping you push. Just like in a physical sport, there are many different techniques available. The L&D nurses around the world bring a wonderful array of personalities to the job, and as such, they have varying approaches to the task at hand.

There's a special alchemy that transpires when the personalities of all the people involved in a delivery mesh and complement one another. If you find that your personality clashes with your nurse, check with the charge nurse and see if there is someone with whom you would perform better. This could be the difference between successful pushing and vaginal delivery and winding up with a cesarean section you didn't want. It's worth asking the question.

Then there's the other half of your dynamic duo: your labor coach or birthing partner. Ideally, by the time you go into labor, you and your partner have done a lot of preparation. You've taken classes, learned how to breathe together, and read this book. Birthing today, more than ever, is a team event.

Your coach need not be your husband or partner; many women have neither, or their mate doesn't feel up to the task. Some moms hire a professional labor coach, often called a doula. One study showed having a doula reduced the cesarean section rate by 45 percent in laboring women. I can't overstress the importance of having excellent support.[IV]

Every mom-to-be is unique. Different people motivate themselves in different ways, and they perform better under different circumstances. This is true in the delivery room, too. The standard American "legs up in stirrups, on your back" stance may not be the best pushing position for everyone. Some women use a squatting bar to help maintain a squat position for pushing. Others push better on their side, with one leg partly raised. Oftentimes, the nurse and the labor partner will actively push the legs back to help open up the pelvic outlet. Just remember to rest your legs between pushes to avoid nerve damage (see Chapter 11 of *The Safe Baby System* for a more detailed discussion on pushing).

Just as your position is important, so is your baby's. The position of the baby during labor can increase your chances for having a cesarean. Classically, when the baby's head is OP—occiput posterior—the head needs to turn, or rotate, into the OA—occiput anterior—position in order to push the baby out. Think of two spoons stacked together. The shape of your pelvis is one spoon. The baby typically needs to bend with the shape of the pelvis—to dip below the pubic bone—in order to come out. That's the OA position: when the baby delivers vaginally, face down, looking toward the rectum.

These are the moments when a nurse's expertise can be incredibly helpful. By positioning you on your side, she may be able to help the baby turn. Ask your nurse for any tricks she may have accumulated over the years. What are the signs of the baby's head being in the OP position? One indication is that once you have an epidural, the contraction pain goes away, but you still have some residual lower back

> **INSIDER SECRET**
>
> If the baby's head stays in the OP position, it is much harder to push the baby out. It's a problem of elemental physics. However, I've certainly witnessed many women push babies out OP. It takes tremendous effort and time, and both you and your OB have to be willing, but it is possible. Be sure to inform your doctor of your wishes beforehand. Take "Cynthia," whose firstborn was in the OP position. Because she was very athletic and in great shape, her OB allowed her to push . . . for 4 hours! In the end, the baby came out just fine—happy and healthy. Of course, after that, Cynthia's second and third children were no sweat!

pain. That's because the baby's head is pressing on the nerves in the posterior pelvis—the lumbo-sacral plexus of nerves. This pain may not be relieved by an epidural of the typical strength, so a stronger concentration may help to relieve the pain, albeit at the expense of having rubbery legs for a while.

Both your nurse and your coaching partner are going to be invaluable to you, suppliers of support, energy, and encouragement. No doubt about it: pushing a baby out is hard work, and you're going to need all the help you can get. If you get an epidural, your body is still doing hard work, even if you don't feel the pain. You've got to think like an athlete to perform like one!

Do what you can to keep your energy up for the home stretch. Try to conserve your energy, and nap when you can. Keep drinking fluids. Many hospitals allow clear fluids—clear broth, clear tea, coffee without milk, apple juice, or sports drinks like Gatorade (some studies show that you have more energy and push better if you consume a sports drink during labor). Some people advocate eating some protein before you go to the hospital, but it may not be a good idea to eat a large meal on the way in; having a full stomach increases your chances for aspirating your food if you end up needing a cesarean section under general anesthesia.

It's not only your energy level that needs to be maintained. Your labor partner's energy level is important, too! They have to be your guardian angel and your watchdog, keeping an eye on you when you are tired or sleeping. Your partner should know as much as you do about what's going to happen. He or she should be completely aware of your medical wishes, making sure that you're getting the correct medications and asking questions when anything seems out of the ordinary. If for whatever reason you aren't cognizant at any point during the delivery, you'll need someone close by who can make decisions on your behalf.

Speeding Up Labor: What You Need to Know

There's a lot of Internet buzz about using Pitocin (oxytocin) during labor. Much of it is not supported by the scientific literature. So let's talk for a moment about what oxytocin does do and what problems to watch out for.

There can be several reasons your OB or midwife may want to start oxytocin. Maybe your contractions are not very frequent. Maybe you're not dilating that fast. Maybe you're having an induction. For any or all of these reasons, your doctor may want to speed things along with your labor. And, like most things, you need to consider the risks and benefits.

Using oxytocin to increase the frequency and strength of your contractions can help you have a successful vaginal delivery and avoid a cesarean. However, it must be used cautiously. Oxytocin must be administered by a carefully controlled infusion pump with a well-working IV. You want to ensure that you are kept on "low dose," not "high dose," oxytocin. Typically, that translates into an infusion of oxytocin starting at 2 milliUnits per minute and increasing by no more than 2 milliUnits per minute every 15-40 minutes.[v]

If your IV is not working well, or if the IV is positional (flows okay if you hold your hand in one position, but not in another), beware. The infusion may be erratic, leading to unsuspected changes in the true delivery rate of the medication. See www.safebabysystem.com/IV for a video showing how to have your IV problem free. And even with a smooth infusion and IV, oxytocin does increase the chances for hyperstimulation of the uterus and fetal decels. When the uterus contracts too frequently or fails to adequately relax during contractions, the baby gets less blood flowing to the placenta and less oxygen. Prompt recognition and treatment is vital if you don't want to end up with a crash cesarean.

Because cervical ripening agents can also cause hyperstimulation of the uterus, resulting in an unhappy baby from being squeezed too much or too often, the nurse or doctor may also remove the prostaglandin medication and give you terbutaline instead. Terbutaline will typically stop the contractions. Hyperstimulation, also called tachysystole, occurs when your uterus is contracting >5 times in 10 min or when the uterus does not fully relax between contractions.[vi]

If you prefer not to add another drug to the cocktail, a Foley catheter balloon may be inserted into the cervix when it first starts to open up. By applying constant mild mechanical pressure within the cervix, it helps to dilate the cervix faster and better than medication alone. By opening up the cervix faster, the success rate of inductions increases, leading to more vaginal deliveries and fewer cesarean sections.

Now let's talk about AROM, another mechanical method of inducing labor. AROM, or artificial rupture of membranes, means the doctor, nurse, or midwife will break the bag of waters (amnion) in order to speed up labor. AROM is generally very safe and affective. However, you have to make sure that the fetal head is well-engaged (low down in pelvis) and not high or floating when they perform the amniotomy. Otherwise, when the bag of waters is ruptured, the umbilical cord can gush out with the amniotic fluid first, causing the baby's head to come down on top of the umbilical cord and pinching off the flow of blood to the baby. Fetal bradycardia (low heart rate) quickly ensues as the blood flow from the placenta to the baby is cut off.

If an AROM is done with the baby's head in the wrong position, the immediate short-term remedy is for someone to push the baby's head up off the umbilical cord with their hand via the vagina. The problem is that then you get taken back for an emergency cesarean, as that position can't be maintained for very long.

Learn to read the fetal monitor strips, the printouts on the monitor in your hospital room. The lower tracing is the contraction pattern. OBs want to see contractions every 2-3 minutes. The external monitor, however, does not actually measure the pressure or strength of the contraction, but merely the timing and duration. That means that a higher peak does not necessarily reflect a stronger contraction.

Often, if the contractions appear frequent enough but you are not dilating according to your OB's plan (typically 1 cm/hour dilation), they may put an IUPC inside of you. An IUPC, or intrauterine pressure catheter, directly measures the pressure within the uterus and medically defines the adequacy of the contraction, measured in Montevideo units. This is especially common for mothers who have chosen to deliver through VBAC.

The downside to this is that the more you have vaginal exams, and the more you have tubes and wires leading up inside of you, the more chance you have for developing infection and a fever called chorioamnionitis. "Chorio," the abbreviation that is more often used, means infection in your uterus and/or placenta. One common pathogen that causes chorio is group B streptococcus, which your OB will routinely check for. Other bacteria that live in the vagina can track up into the uterus causing infection. Chorio typically occurs when you have fever, fetal tachycardia (fast heart rate: >160 BPM), and tenderness in the uterus. Chorio requires treatment with strong antibiotics, typically ampicillin and gentamicin, when first diagnosed.[vi] Your baby may need a couple of days of antibiotics too.

Other events that can lead to increased chance of infection include poor sterile techniques with IVs, multiple vaginal exams, internal monitors, and "bad" strains of bacteria that colonize your colon, vagina, and uterus. If you have signs of vaginal infection during your pregnancy, be sure to tell your OB so that you can receive prompt and effective treatment. You'll decrease your chance for preterm birth as well as infection of the uterus during or after delivery. More on this in the next chapter.

Prolonged labor, oxytocin use, and infection all increase the risk for uterine atony—a "lazy uterus" that doesn't want to contract after delivery. More on uterine atony in Part II.

* * *

When you're in labor, remember to keep the lines of communication open with your OB or midwife. She's there to answer any questions you may have. If she feels that a vaginal delivery is no longer safe and that you need a C-section, you are entitled to ask why. You may also ask:

- Is it safe for me to wait longer?

- Is it safe for the baby to wait longer?

- What are the risks involved with waiting?

- Are my contractions adequate?

- Am I pushing well?

- Is there anything I can do to help avoid a cesarean?

The more you know, the better chance you'll be having your baby on *your* terms. Ultimately your Obstetrician is the expert you have chosen to help you birth and is the final authority as to whether you need a cesarean and how fast it needs to be performed. Remember to pick one you trust and you feel you can work together with. In the heat of the moment is NOT the time to disagree.

And if you've decided, either by choice or necessity, to have a cesarean, rest assured: the ball is still in your court. To ensure that you and your baby have a safe, healthy delivery, keep reading.

Things To Keep In Mind

- Learn the language of cesareans, so you know what's going on in the delivery room.

- Epidurals do not cause C-sections.

- In addition to the delivery room team, it's great to have your own partner or coach – a nurse, a doula, a midwife, or your husband.

- Keep up your energy during labor – frequent sips of clear liquids, rest when you can.

- Oxytocin can increase the frequency and strength of your contractions and help you have a successful vaginal delivery and avoid a cesarean. However, it must be used cautiously.

- Know what questions to ask your OB or midwife as labor goes forward and especially when they start talking about needing a cesarean.

Go to **www.SafeBabySystem.com/bonus** for additional information.

REFERENCES

[i] ACOG committee opinion Number 326, December 2005 Inappropriate Use of the Terms Fetal Distress and Birth Asphyxia.

[ii] ACOG Practice Bulletin 116, Management of Intrapartum Fetal Heart Rate Tracings, November 2010.)

[iii] ACOG Committee Opinion No. 339, June 2006 – Analgesia and Cesarean Delivery Rates, Reaffirmed 2008.

[iv] McGrath SK. Birth 2008:35:92-97. A randomized controlled trial of continuous labor support for middle-class couples: effect on Cesarean delivery rates.

[v] ACOG Practice Bulletin, NUMBER 107, AUGUST 2009 Induction of Labor.

[vi] Robinson B, Nelson L. A Review of the Proceedings from the 2008 NICHD Workshop on Standardized Nomenclature for Cardiotocography Update on Definitions, Interpretative Systems With Management Strategies, and Research Priorities in Relation to Intrapartum Electronic Fetal Monitoring
Rev Obstet Gynecol. 2008:1:186-192.

[vii] Marrazzo JM. Evolving issues in understanding and treating bacterial vaginosis. Expert Review of Antiinfective Therapy 2004;2: 913–22.

PART II

PREPARE FOR

and

HAVING A CESAREAN

Additional Bonus Materials are being created just for you.
As a special thank you, go to
www.SafeBabySystem.com/bonus

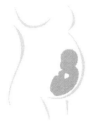

Chapter 4

During Pregnancy: Doing the Leg Work

So, you're having a cesarean. Don't worry! In Part II, I'm going to share with you everything you need to know so that you and your baby are just fine before, during, and after your delivery.

A C-section gives you the gift of life. However, it's important to remember that it is still surgery. And surgery is serious business. It's nothing to be scared of; it's just something to be educated about. The more you can learn and participate, the better off you are. And yes— you, the patient, can actually help us, the caregivers, take better care of you. As Tom Cruise says in *Jerry Maguire*: "Help me help you."

In the last chapter, we briefly discussed the role of your nurse and your labor partner, particularly in the context of a vaginal delivery. In the following chapters, I'm going to introduce you to the rest of the cast—all the people who will be helping you during your surgery. Then we'll go over all the risks you need to be aware of so that if you find yourself in a scary situation, you'll be able to think clearly and choose wisely, having already discussed the options in depth. I'll also share with you the insider tricks and secrets that make surviving cesarean a piece of cake. You can not only survive a C-section; you can thrive during the birth of your child.

Your work begins in the nine months leading up to your big day.

Staying in Shape

In Chapter 2, we talked about keeping yourself healthy in order to have a vaginal delivery. If you're having a C-section, you're not off the hook! Maintaining your health is just as important for you, if not more so. Cesarean—just like any surgery—is an invasive procedure and hence is traumatic for the human body. In order for your body to heal and recover from surgery, you need to be nutritionally fit, in good shape, and have a great attitude.

First and foremost: nutrition. Your body uses the building blocks you give it to function, perform, and repair itself. That's why maintaining a healthy diet and taking your vitamins is plain common sense. Choose foods with a low glycemic index, drink lots of pure water, and eat organic whenever you can.

And don't forget to take your vitamins. Did you know that vitamin C and the amino acids proline and lysine are used to make the connective tissue framework throughout the body? That's pretty important when you're having surgery.[i] Vitamins and minerals are key co-factors in innumerable processes within your body. They not only build your body into a strong fortress for your baby; they help build a healthy baby, too.

There's another, relatively new star on the nutritional stage: probiotics. Like it or not, your body is colonized by trillions upon trillions of bacteria. Some are friendly, while many are not.

Ever wonder why a surprising number of people these days, both women and men, have "sensitive stomachs"? Eating certain foods sends them fleeing to the bathroom, complaining of GI distress, bloating,

---

INSIDER SECRET

Here's a suggested daily dose as part of your prenatal vitamins:
- 1000 mcg Folate
- 1000 mg DHA (a type of fish oil)
- 1000 mg vitamin C
- A probiotic supplement

For further information on vitamins and what foods to eat during pregnancy, see Chapter 4 of *The Safe Baby System.*

---

and diarrhea. The problem is that the good bacteria—the kind that are supposed to be our symbiotic co-hosts—are not the most frequent dwellers anymore. Changes in farming methods, the way we eat, what we eat, antibiotic usage in people and animals, high-sugar diets, and lifestyle changes all contribute to why we no longer have the same predominant groups of beneficial bacteria. This shift in the bacterial balance of our bodies has wreaked havoc on our intestines.

When you get an infection, your white blood cells will come and fight off the bad guys—the bacteria that causes diseases. However, you can decrease your chance for infections by being stocked up on the good bacteria, also known as probiotics.

These good bacteria do not cause diseases in humans. Even better, they crowd out or even kill the bad bacteria. As you prepare for a C-section, infection is *not* your friend. There is always a higher risk of infection during surgery, so you want to do everything in your power to ward off the bad kind of bacteria and invite the good kind in. Pregnant women with vaginal infections (bacterial vaginosis) have a higher risk for miscarriage, chorioamnionitis, premature rupture of the amniotic membranes, preterm birth, and postpartum endometritis (infection of the uterus).[ii]

Probiotics aren't just important for you; they're important for your baby. Where does your baby get colonized by the good bacteria? From Mom, of course! Many studies have shown the benefits to the baby when mom takes the good bacteria. Your baby can even pick up the good bacteria on the way out of the birth canal. That may be why children born by cesarean have a higher rate of allergic rhinocon-junctivitis (runny nose) and asthma by 24 percent.[iii] The bacteria in your baby's intestine actually affect their immune systems and T-helper cell function.

Changes in the intestinal bacteria flora have also been associated with sensitization to food allergens. A recent review found evidence of increased risk of food allergies in children delivered by C-section.[iv] This is all the more reason to combat these possible effects by taking probiotics during pregnancy. It will help keep you safe from infection and keep your baby free of allergies and asthma. There has even been some evidence to show that taking probiotics can reduce premature births. There's little risk, so why not? Stock up on the good guys and your baby will thank you.

Physical activity is next in the trinity of good preparation. Exercising sets a precedent for your body to heal itself. When you're in good physical shape, your body simply tolerates physical stress better, meaning you pop back from exercise more quickly. The same goes for surgery: the better shape you're in, the quicker you'll bounce back after surgery. I've seen it in thousands of men and women who've had all kinds of surgery: the better shape you're in, the faster you move around, bounce back, and recover.

INSIDER SECRET

Another factor that affects how well you heal from a C-section is age. I promised to tell it like it is, so here goes: as you get older, you heal more slowly. This is because certain crucial hormones in your body decrease as you age—the ones related to stress and repair, unfortunately. Growth hormone, testosterone, and DHEA all start decreasing after your twenties. Obviously, changing your age isn't really an option. But if you're over the 40-year mark, be sure to get a full medical check-up from your internist.

I remember "Tom," a very athletic man, who underwent a hip replacement. He was up and about, walking around the very next day! He even amazed his surgeon and the company that makes the equipment. They wanted to know what he did differently than all the other patients. To me it was obvious: he was younger than most people who have hip surgery, and he was in great shape. His muscles and tendons were able to hold the leg and hip in correct alignment. Tom could have been the "poster child" for hip surgery!

The same rule applies to moms. The women who recover the fastest from a C-section are the athletes. That doesn't mean you have to be a professional athlete—you can still have a great recovery, even without any Olympic medals on the shelf. My suggestion is that you start immediately with some type of moderate exercise. Running, yoga, swimming, and even walking all fit the bill.

We've talked about how obesity leads to an increased cesarean section rate. It also leads to complications from surgery. In other words, obesity doesn't just increase your chances of needing a C-section; it increases your chances for trouble once you've had one! Risks include infection, wound dehiscence (breakdown), difficult anesthesia placement, higher mortality from general anesthesia, and higher chance of blood clots in the legs, pelvic veins, and lungs. All the more reason to get obesity in check as soon as you can.

Then there's the attitude part of the equation. The shape you're in emotionally during your pregnancy is just as important as your physical prowess. Emotional stress can start from many sources—relationships, work, difficulty getting pregnant, and mixed feelings about having a baby. No feeling is "wrong." What's important is that you express your feelings and work through them.

Talk to a close friend or a professional. A qualified therapist can work wonders in helping you walk through some of your fear and anxiety. Many women find yoga and meditation helpful in calming their minds. Hypnosis recordings can also help. Don't knock it until you've tried it— an accomplished friend of mine is a hypnotherapist who has helped thousands of people lead productive, stress-free lives. Remember: stress releases hormones that adversely affect your health and the health of your baby, so do what you can to eliminate stress from your mind and body. For additional information see www.SafeBabySystem.com

Your psychology of birthing will have an important role in how fast you recover. The more well-read and well-prepared you are, the better you'll be able to paint mental images of a speedy recovery. A little interior decorating never hurt, either; when you pack for the hospital, be sure to include a few objects that will personalize your hospital room and make you feel good. A picture of a favorite pet or your family can work wonders—anything to brighten your spirits and elevate your mood. And be sure to bring your favorite pillow! Hospital pillows are plastic so they can be cleaned and sanitized between patients, but they don't feel very good to sleep on. Trust me, I know—I've been using them for over twenty years. Some women like to bring their favorite soft blanket too.

Picking Your Hospital

We talked about choosing a hospital in the context of avoiding a cesarean. Not let's discuss how to choose a hospital when you *want* a C-section—or when you and your doctor have decided it's the safest choice for you.

Many people blindly go to the hospital their OB or surgeon prefers. I strongly suggest you do some research and make your own decision. Picking the right place to have your surgery is one of the most important decisions you will make.

While some moms like the idea of a smaller hospital because it seems they will get better, more personalized care, sometimes the exact opposite is true. Because many small hospitals have fewer staff and support services, you may actually *not* get the attention you desire, or worse—the attention you need. I usually encourage women to seek out larger hospitals because they have more people on staff 24/7, a larger selection of specialized services, and more reserves in the blood bank.

In general, a hospital that only delivers 1,000 babies per year is a low-volume hospital. Once you get above 2,000 deliveries per year, you should be okay. That means there is a large enough volume of deliveries, both vaginal and cesarean, that most emergency services will probably be present. Once you get to ten or more deliveries a day—about 4,000 a year or above—the hospital is high-volume. All the tertiary care staff and services you might need should be readily available.

What are the tools and services you might need in a pinch? X-ray, CT scan, and MRI are all possible. Rapid transfusion of multiple units of blood (PRBC, the red stuff) and specialized clotting (Factor VII concentrate) might also be needed in an emergency. And a specialist at the hospital could help with a complication of surgery, someone like a urologist, neurosurgeon, or infectious disease specialist.

Be sure to ask the following three questions at every hospital you visit:

- What is your C-section rate?

- What is your hemorrhage rate?

- What is your hysterectomy rate?

Conveniently, more and more of this information is posted online. You can check out hospital information at various websites, including www.hospitalcompare.hhs.gov and www.ahrq.gov.

Some specialized questions that may not be listed on a website but that you'll definitely want to ask are:

- Do you have a dedicated, 24/7 staff for L&D, including scrub tech, anesthesiologist, CRNA, OB resident or attending backup, and x-ray specialist? (See Chapter 10 of *The Safe Baby System* for a detailed list of all the people who may be involved in your cesarean delivery.)

- In case of severe bleeding, do you have advanced therapies available like Factor VII concentrate or Cell Saver?

- How many units of FFP (fresh frozen plasma) do you typically have "in stock" for emergencies? Or do you have to call the Red Cross for supply during a major hemorrhage?

You'll probably opt for spinal or epidural anesthesia, but in case a general anesthesia is required, you also want to ask the following questions:

- In case of difficult intubation, what extra specialized equipment do you have *immediately* available in Labor & Delivery?

- Do you have some form of emergency airway equipment— LMA, fiberoptic bronchoscope for intubation, transtracheal jet ventilation, cricothyrotomy kit, etc.?

- How many anesthesiologists (physicians) or nurse anesthetists do you have in the hospital? Who do they call if they need help? And how far away are they? Upstairs or at home?

Never feel like you're asking too many questions. *These questions can save your life and the life of your baby.*

An Embolism: Your Worst Enemy

As you prepare for your cesarean delivery, it's important that you know the three biggest risks to your own health and safety: hemorrhage, preeclampsia, and embolism. The bad news is that the Big Three are the leading causes of maternal death. The good news is that there is plenty you can do to improve your odds.

We've already discussed preeclampsia as it pertains to avoiding a C-section, and we'll take a closer look at hemorrhage in Chapter 7 when we talk about recovery. Right now I want to discuss the third danger, and the one that occurs before, during or after surgery: embolism.

An embolism occurs when an object travels through the bloodstream and causes a blockage of a blood vessel. There are many different kinds of embolisms, including air (entrainment of air into the veins of the uterus during a cesarean section), amniotic fluid (fetal cells and other compounds floating around in the amniotic fluid) and thrombotic (blood clot). Embolism is the most deadly of the Big Three and kills more women today than any other cause.[vii] Fortunately, you can take some steps to significantly reduce your chances for these problems.

Air Embolism

During a C-section, if you entrain a large amount of air into your veins, you can get an "air lock" blocking the passage of blood through the heart. Based on experiments, the amount of air needed to do this in humans is fairly large—close to 60 ml. A tiny air bubble that you sometimes see in your IV line is less than 0.5 ml and shouldn't harm you.

However, if you have a hole in your heart, most commonly a probe patent foramen ovale, then it is possible for a relatively smaller amount of air to enter the vein, go to the right side of the heart, cross the wall in your atrium via the hole, and enter the left side of the heart. The left side of the heart pumps the oxygenated blood into your arteries and to the rest of the body. If air enters your arteries, even a relatively small amount, it could occlude flow through that artery, causing a lack of oxygen to that part of the brain and possibly even a stroke.

Almost 15 percent of people have a probe patent foramen ovale, but far fewer actually have routine flow through the hole. Still, better to be safe than sorry. If you know you have a patent foramen ovale, tell your OB, nurse, and anesthesiologist. Also, ask for an air filter added to your IV line to ensure that no air can enter your IV and go to your heart or brain. In fact don't just ask—insist on it.

Most health care workers aren't too worried about this possibility. Even if you *do* have a small air bubble enter your vein, the normal path takes it to the right side of your heart—atrium, ventricle, and then lungs—which would essentially filter it out, thereby protecting you. However, being educated and looking out for number one (you!) is an important part of surviving your cesarean with flying colors.

Amniotic Fluid Embolism

Fortunately, an amniotic fluid embolism (AFE) is considered rare, occurring in 1/6000 deliveries. Unfortunately, it has a 50 percent mortality rate. This type of embolism occurs most commonly during rapid cervical dilation, when the veins in the endocervix can tear, allowing amniotic fluid into the blood stream, and during cesarean section, when amniotic fluid can enter the bloodstream directly through the cut in the uterus.

Interestingly, amniotic fluid and fetal cells can commonly be found in small amounts in mom's blood. Hence the occurrence of an AFE doesn't just have to do solely with the amount that enters the blood, but the quality of the prostaglandins and other vasoactive compounds that might be present in the amniotic fluid.

How can you make a difference in such a rare and fatal occurrence? Picking a large, well-known hospital can be helpful, ideally a hospital that has a lot of resources—people, equipment, and blood banking that can be activated at a moment's notice. Also, know the signs and symptoms of AFE: sudden hypotension (feeling lightheaded or faint) and cardiovascular collapse (passing out, very low blood pressure), shortness of breath, hypoxia (deprivation of oxygen supply), fetal bradycardia (low fetal heart rate), DIC (a type of blood clotting/bleeding disorder), and seizures.

In my years as an OB Anesthesiologist, I've personally seen a couple of pregnant women with AFE. With immediate recognition, prompt and very aggressive treatment—and perhaps a dash of luck—these moms have walked out of the hospital with a healthy newborn in their arms.

Thrombotic Embolism

Thrombotic embolism occurs when a blood clot goes from your leg or pelvis to your heart and lungs. Of the three types of embolism, this is the one on which you can have the greatest (and easiest) impact in the months leading up to your delivery.

Pregnancy brings a lot of changes to your body. One of the things that changes is your blood. When you're pregnant, you have a slightly lower concentration of red cells, the kind that carry oxygen around, but a higher concentration of the proteins in your blood that help you to form blood clots. The body was probably designed this way to help you form blood clots after delivery, reducing the chance of hemorrhaging to death. Remember, in the pre-medical days, one in fifteen women died during childbirth. Thank goodness we live in the era of epidurals and blood banking!

This may help save your life during delivery, but also increases the formation of blood clots in your body, especially your legs. If the blood clot grows in size, it can become a DVT—deep venous thrombosis. One study from Canada showed the rate of deep vein thrombosis (DVT) at 12.1/10,000 births and pulmonary embolism (PE) at 5.4/10,000 births.[viii] With DVT, a particularly bad clot can sometimes dislodge and travel to your heart and lungs. A very large embolism to the heart, called a saddle embolism, can block all blood flow through the heart. That's something you definitely *don't* want.

And it's something that can easily be prevented. Knowing the signs, symptoms, and preemptive actions will dramatically decrease your chances of an embolism. First off, do a little research on your family tree. Do you or anyone in your family have a history of blood clots? What about pregnancy loss? As it turns out, a common reason for recurrent pregnancy loss is small genetic variations that can further increase your tendency to form blood clots. What probably happens is that clots form around the placenta, cutting off flow and resulting in loss of the pregnancy.

Second: watch for leg swelling. Yes, some swelling is common in pregnancy, but the swelling should be equal on both sides. If one leg starts to become larger, or if you experience tenderness, pain, and redness, call your doctor immediately. You might also feel a tough string or "cord" in your leg. These are all signs of a blood clot in your leg. And if you heed the call, you'll still have time to catch it early and treat it before it grows large enough to be a life-threatening danger to you or your baby.

More ominous signs that the blood clot has traveled to the lungs include sudden onset of SOB (shortness of breath) and decrease in your blood oxygen level. You might also feel like your heart is racing. Obviously, these are pretty non-specific symptoms, but if you experience any of them, call your doctor right away. You might need a special kind of CT scan called a spiral CT to detect a pulmonary embolism.

Being alert to these problems can literally mean the difference between life and death. I remember a situation where self-awareness, education, and proper action literally saved a woman's life. "Carly" was a young woman, very slender and physically active, whose pregnancy was proceeding uneventfully until she felt something in her leg. Carly's calf grew very tender, and it was getting worse. Because she was an avid runner, Carly thought she had torn a muscle exercising. But after two days, when she could no longer walk on the leg, she called her doctor.

In the hospital, the ultrasound confirmed that she had a blood clot in her leg. Carly received heparin treatment and got better. Three months later, she had similar symptoms, this time further up her leg. She immediately called her doctor, who called her in for a checkup. On the way to see him, she experienced shortness of breath. During her work-up, the hospital staff discovered that she had one of those genetic variants that increases your tendency to clot (known as hypercoaguability). She was treated with the right medication and is now permanently on a 'blood thinner' (anti-coagulant) so that her blood will not clot as well.

Carly delivered her firstborn by C-section two years ago, and both she and her son are doing just fine. Because Carly knew the symptoms and went directly to the hospital, she got the right diagnosis and received appropriate therapy, paving the way for a smooth delivery and a healthy future. Her alertness probably saved her life.

* * *

The alertness that you cultivate during your pregnancy will serve you well during delivery. Now let's talk about how to ensure that you're alert, aware, and educated on "D Day" (Delivery Day) . . . or rather, C-Day. The day of your C-section.

Things To Keep In Mind

- A C-section is surgery, but it's nothing to be scared of; it's just something to be educated about.

- Proper nutrition and supplementation, including probiotics, are essential for your health throughout pregnancy.

- Physical exercise and activity, along with stress reduction, make your pregnancy easier and your C-section safer.

- Many people blindly go to the hospital their OB or insurance company prefers. I strongly suggest you do some research and make your own decision.

- The three biggest risks to your own health and safety: hemorrhage, preeclampsia, and embolism. You can be reduce some of the risks by taking proper care of yourself during pregnancy.

- Large hospitals are generally better equipped to cope with complications like embolisms and hemorrhage to keep them from causing fatalities.

- Pregnancy changes many things in your body, including your blood.

- Leg swelling could be indicative of a blood clot and should be taken extremely seriously.

Go to **www.SafeBabySystem.com/bonus** for additional information.

REFERENCES

[i] Ivanov V et al. Anti-atherogenic effects of a mixture of ascorbic acid, lysine, proline, arginine, cysteine, and green tea phenolics in human aortic smooth muscle cells. J Cardiovasc Pharmacol 2007:49:140-145.

[ii] Marrazzo JM. Evolving issues in understanding and treating bacterial vaginosis. Expert Rev Anti Infect Ther. 2004 Dec; 2(6):913-22. And Trenev N. Probiotics: nature's internal healers. Avery Publishing Group. Garden City Park, NY 1998.

[iii] Renz-Polster H. Clin Exp Allergy 2005:35:1466-72. Caesarean section delivery and the risk of allergic disorders in childhood.

[iv] Koplin J. Pediatr Allergy Immunol 2008:19:682-7. Is caesarean delivery associated with sensitization to food allergens and IgE-mediated food allergy: A systematic review.

[v] Reid G, Bocking A. The potential for probiotics to prevent bacterial vaginosis and preterm labor. Am J Obstet Gynecol 2003:189:1202-8. And = Trenev N. Probiotics: Nature's Internal Healers, Avery Publishing Garden City 1998.

[vi] Khan KS et al. WHO analysis of causes of maternal death: a systematic review. Lancet 2006:367:1066.

[vii] CDC MMWR, Pregnancy-Related mortality surveillance – United States, 1991-1999, MMWR Surveillance summaries, February 21, 2003/52(SS02);1-8.

[viii] Liu S et al. Epidemiology of pregnancy associated venous thromboembolism: a population-based study in Canada. J Obstet Gynaecol Can 2009:31:611-20.

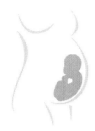

Chapter 5

Pre-Op: Settling In and Hooking Up

I t never fails to amaze me how many misperceptions about surgery persist. Some people think they can show up in the morning of their surgery, having done no preparation whatsoever, and it'll be smooth sailing from there on out. As you've probably picked up by now, I don't buy it for a second. After all: good preparation is at the core of this book, not to mention at the heart of a healthy delivery.

While cesarean sections may be on the rise, they are still a surgery, and just like any other surgery, your success will depend on how well you prepare. When it comes to pre-operative preparation, there's a LOT you can do to ensure your own safety—from taking care of personal hygiene before you leave the house to getting ready for the IV in your hospital room. In this chapter we'll talk about how you can best assist the medical staff as you prepare for your cesarean so that you are no longer a passive patient, but an active participant in your own care.

Personal Grooming

You no doubt want to look your best for all the pictures you'll be taking of you and your newborn. These are the pictures you will treasure forever. Just remember: safety comes first! And though it may not have crossed your mind, your personal grooming—jewelry, nails, shaving, and skin care—does come into play when you're having a cesarean. It all starts at home.

Let's talk about jewelry. The problem with jewelry is that it's metal, and metal conducts electricity. During your cesarean, just like during any other surgery, the OB uses some type of electrosurgical unit or ESU, commonly referred to as the "Bovie," to cut through the tissue layers. By burning and cutting at the same time, the Bovie passes an intense current through a pinpoint area of your body to produce enough heat to cut the tissue and simultaneously cauterize it to seal the wound and reduce the bleeding. To do so, the electricity always has to form a circuit, or circle. If you put electric current in one place, it has to come out somewhere else. That's why they put a Bovie pad (electrical return pad) on you.

If you are wearing metal jewelry, it could form another possible path for the electricity to return, resulting in a burn. So no jewelry allowed during surgery! It's easier to Photoshop the jewelry into place once than to cover up a burn spot forever.

Then there's the issue of makeup. Back in the old days and before some of the latest technology, we used to depend on looking at your skin color to see if you were pink (well-oxygenated) or blue (low oxygen and a sign of trouble). I'm a little old school in my method—I prefer it if the woman isn't wearing so much makeup that I can't tell her true skin color. Many of today's doctors and nurses don't have the old-time clinical framework, and they won't hassle you about it.

Still, I suggest keeping your makeup light. When people aren't feeling well, they often develop pallor. Have you ever been told you were white as a sheet when you were ill? That's because your body is no longer perfusing your skin with an adequate amount of blood to maintain that healthy, rosy color. If you're losing blood after a C-section, it's helpful for the doctor to be able to read the signs from your face (as well as more technical systems of measurement). This 'old school' trick has helped me to catch trends early many times—helping both of us!

If you receive general anesthesia, many anesthesiologists use a brain wave monitor to help determine if you are deeply asleep or not. But you need good skin contact with the electrodes, so they will first clean your forehead with alcohol swabs. It may be worth it to forgo the heavy foundation, because your anesthesiologist is probably going to take it off your forehead as a part of the pre-op anyway.

I've seen a lot of women who come in for their elective cesarean looking fresh and fabulous—hair, makeup, nails all done. Again, this is up to you. But here's a tip regarding your nails: if you're going to have them done, please use a clear or light color. Being able to see the color of your nail beds is an important clinical sign of oxygenation and perfusion.

A required monitor used during all surgeries is called a pulse oximeter, which measures the oxygen in your blood by putting a special light through your fingernail. The technology for the pulse oximeter has gotten pretty good—most of them can still get a reading, no matter what color your nails—but the dark polishes may still interfere with a correct measurement. Avoid blue and black colors in particular, as these cause the most interference. Who wants to depend solely on technology rendered iffy when your life may depend on it? Play it safe and keep the color light or clear. You'll still look beautiful.

Infection is also something you want to be wary of during the pre-op stage. In spite of all the fancy new antibiotics—and often because of them—infections can be worse than ever. The new and evolved type of infection is perhaps the most menacing of all: the drug-resistant kind. This kind of bacteria and possible infection thrives in hospitals. Infections following a cesarean typically occur in 3-5 percent of women.[i]

There are several pre-op steps you can take to decrease your chances of getting an infection during your surgery and hospital stay. First, start out with the right bacteria. We talked in the last chapter about probiotics, which eliminate the bad bacteria that cause bacterial vaginosis and enodometritis after surgery.[ii] Step one is preventative: make friendly bacteria a normal part of your healthy living so that they can outcompete the bad bacteria you may encounter during your pregnancy and C-section.

The second step is to get rid of the bad bacteria by cleansing them before surgery. And I'm not talking about a colon cleanse; I mean thoroughly cleansing your skin. It goes without saying that the hospital staff appreciates it if you shower and bathe before your surgery. But in addition to using normal soap, you can actually wash yourself with something that keeps the bacteria count on your skin down, and often kills bacteria completely.

I learned this one from a famous cardiac surgeon in New York. He often performed long, complex open-heart surgeries. Of course all his patients had the usual surgical scrub around the skin incision, and they all received copious amounts of antibiotics. Yet he took it one step further. This surgeon had all of his patients shower and scrub themselves with CHG, chlorhexidine gluconate, a potent antibacterial compound. The CHG antiseptic sticks to the skin and provides a prolonged anti-bacterial effect. This one simple technique significantly reduced the number of post-op infections in his patients. Smart guy!

As it turns out, this surgeon was way ahead of the game. Twenty years later, the old iodine-based surgical scrub has lost favor and the newer alcohol-chlorhexidine scrub has been proven to be far more effective. Now chlorhexidine is sold over the counter in drug stores, and you can take the same preemptive measures yourself by using CHG to clean your body before your cesarean.

Now let's talk about shaving. The nurse will wind up shaving your pubic hair very low, so that there is no hair near the incision area for your cesarean. However, studies have shown that when you shave

---

INSIDER SECRET

Having asked many women with outstanding skin *their* secrets over the years, I've noticed a trend. Many of the women who had the best skin used some olive-oil-based product, rubbing it in daily. They also drank a lot of pure water. Could it be that simple?

immediately before surgery, the chance for skin infection is increased. That's because when you shave, you create little tiny cuts in the skin. These tiny cuts actually increase the access of bacteria into the skin, the first step toward a skin infection.

You are far better off shaving yourself, or waxing if you prefer, the day before your C-section, so your skin is uncut and uncompromised at the time of surgery. You can also use clippers, which don't actually contact or cut the skin. Many hospitals now use clippers to reduce skin infections. Clippers don't remove hair completely, but leave a slight stubble on your skin.

Speaking of your skin: take good care of it. Drink lots of pure clean water, something I always advocate. Most women also use some kind of moisturizer—you probably have a favorite brand. I know some women who use simple organic olive oil! Good skin care is important in avoiding dry, cracked skin, as dry skin makes you susceptible to skin infections. Healthy skin not only looks good; it heals faster.

Hospital-grade soap is the harsher, antibacterial kind, which is typically tough on the skin. Also, hospital air is very dry. This keeps down the proliferation of bacteria and mold, but it can also be tough on the nose and skin. Bring some moisturizer—your body will thank you.

Here's another tip. So many women complain to me about their dry lips. The dryness of the hospital air, mixed with increased breathing during labor, will often result in dry, cracked lips after delivery. Bring Vaseline, Chapstick, or your favorite lip gloss to keep your lips moist. Not only will it feel better—you'll look great for those family pictures, too.

INSIDER SECRET

When you moisturize, be sure to leave a 4"x8" spot on the outside of your thigh for the Bovie pad. I've seen women who used so much oil that their skin was slippery. This makes it hard for the Bovie pad to stick, reducing the electrical return surface area and increasing the chance for a burn on your skin.

Now you're all groomed and ready for your trip to the hospital. What next? Putting a game plan into action for once you're there.

Once You've Arrived

The first thing you'll do when you come to Labor & Delivery is check in. This process varies a bit from hospital to hospital, but every institution generally has the same type of paperwork. It helps to have pre-registered so that you've been assigned a medical record number. During registration you'll give your insurance information and an ID like a driver's license. This is also when many women first find out what is covered by your insurance, and what is not covered.

INSIDER SECRET

Even if you're going to a preferred hospital for your insurance, some services are NOT included in the main hospital bill. Sometimes an individual physician's services, such as a radiologist, anesthesiologist, an infectious disease specialist, will not be included on your insurance plan. It definitely pays to check this out ahead of time.

When you get past the admissions process, your nurse will start doing your paperwork. You should always keep a copy of your medical history, including your obstetric history, with you during the second half of your pregnancy. While the hospital should have a copy of your pre-natal record from your OB's office, sometimes it disappears into the black hole of paperwork, never to be seen again. And in the off chance that something happens to you while you are not near the hospital where you're scheduled for a C-section, it's important that there not be any guessing or filling in the gaps of your medical history.

In your personal medical history, don't forget to include any surgeries you have had. Be sure to document anyone in your family who has had trouble with anesthesia. One item specific to pregnancy is whether you have been tested for Group B Streptococcus (GBS status) colonization in your vagina, an infection that can spread to the baby and which requires treatment with antibiotics before you deliver in order to prevent that from happening. If you are positive for GBS, you will typically be treated with ampicillin or penicillin.

If you have asthma, you are probably pretty well-tuned to your disease. Pregnancy can improve asthma or make it worse. Usually, if your asthma got better with pregnancy, it won't be a problem at delivery. And if you've been pregnant before and didn't experience any problems, you're in the clear; what happens in one pregnancy predicts how your body will respond in the next one. Many asthmatics use a bronchodilating inhaler, such as albuterol, on an as-needed basis. The hospital can give you one, or—even better—a "breathing treatment" by a respiratory therapist.

I'm an advocate for a hospital-administered nebulizer breathing treatment. Studies have shown that when people use their handheld inhaler, they actually inhale only a fraction of the intended dose of medication. The hospital nebulizer, on the other hand, generates a fine mist that you can inhale deeply into your lungs without having to time your breathing or even do anything different. The mist is comprised of much smaller droplets that easily carry themselves all the way down into your lungs with a simple breath. One prophylactic breathing treatment can prevent trouble later. As the saying goes, "An ounce of prevention is worth a pound of cure."

Be sure to tell your nurse and anesthesiologist about ALL your allergies, not just about any allergies to medicines. The more everyone taking care of you knows about you, the safer you are. Especially make sure to include allergies to foods. There can be cross-reaction to certain medications, or more likely the solution the medication is in. Many women say they are allergic to local anesthetic they got at the dentist. Yet, when questioned, the symptoms they felt were heart racing, which is actually due to the absorption of adrenalin in the local anesthetic and is quite a normal response. Another common food allergy that may cross-react with medications include egg and soybeans, which are part of the white liquid medication propofol, an agent commonly used in anesthesia. Some people are even sensitive or allergic to the type of tape used on the skin, for IVs and bandages e.g. cloth tape.

Know your medicines and keep a consummate list with you at all times. This list should include the names, doses, and how often you take them. Or how often you *don't* take them when you're supposed to! Very frequently when I interview patients before surgery, they cannot tell me the correct name or dose of their medicine. Mispronouncing the name may lead to medication errors, as a nurse or doctor may confuse them with similar-sounding medicines. That's why having it all in writing is best.

Full disclosure is of the essence. That means also telling your OB and anesthesiologist about any over-the-counter medications, herbal preparations, or homeopathics you are taking. Include any vitamins, minerals, or fish oils that you are currently taking. Some of the "harmless" preparations can have significant interactions with certain anesthetics or medications. For example, licorice or licorice root, which is now offered as vitamin supplement, may increase your blood pressure and swelling, while ginger and garlic may increase your tendency to bleed.[iii]

It's also your responsibility to tell your doctors if you are sick. No one likes to have to reschedule anything, much less having a baby. But if you have a cold or fever, *please* let your doctor know. It would be safer for you, the staff, and other pregnant women and babies if you stayed home until you got better. If you have a cold or upper respiratory infection, your chance for having a complication from anesthesia and surgery such as pneumonia increases. And if you have a bad cough, watch out. When you cough, you jiggle your belly and even your uterus, making it harder for your OB to sew you back up.

Settling In

So you've made it past the intake desk and are settling into your hospital room. Great! Now let's talk about what you need to know about those pre-op hours.

First rule of the day: ultrasound. If you are having a cesarean for breech presentation, the staff should definitely do a quick ultrasound to check the position of the baby's head before they operate. Just feeling your belly is not 100 percent reliable. There have certainly been times where, to the OB's surprise, he's doing a cesarean for breech and then pulls the baby out head first!

If you're having a repeat cesarean section, an ultrasound is especially important for the OB to know the location of the placenta. If the placenta is "low-anterior," then it's probably in the exact location where the prior cesarean took place, greatly increasing your chances for a placenta accreta. This is because when you have prior surgery on the uterus, you heal and develop some scar tissue, just like you can see on the skin. If the placenta implants inside the uterus on top of a scar, the tissue layers are not normal, and the placenta can implant deeper than normal. By her fourth cesarean, a woman's overall chance of winding up with a hysterectomy is over 2 percent.[iv] This is good to know—forewarned is forearmed.

Second rule of the day: NPO! Nothing Per Oral—or nothing in your mouth. That means no food or drink. The rules on this have become more liberal in recent years; it used to be no food or even water for at least eight hours prior to elective surgery (for emergency surgery, of course, this can't be helped). Today, however, for most types of surgery, the rules have been eased to no solid food for six to eight hours, no clear liquids (apple juice without pulp, sports drinks, water, or even tea or coffee without milk) for four hours, and water in moderation for up to two hours before surgery.[v]

These are just guidelines and, as such, they're not universally mandated. Check with your local hospital, surgeon, or anesthesiologist, and follow the pre-op instructions that they give you very closely.

There's one fluid that breaks the NPO rule, and this is the one that the doctors give you. This is Bicitra, a non-particulate antacid of sodium citrate. Bicitra is given 30 minutes (or less) before your anesthetic to ensure your stomach contents are not acidic in case of aspiration. The drink is rather tart to most women. I suggest taking it like a shot of alcohol—fast. Sometimes serving Bicitra "on the rocks" (with ice chips) also helps dampen the strong tart flavor.

INSIDER SECRET

If you are going to throw up, turn your head to the side. The anesthesiologist should give you a container, usually called a kidney basin (a plastic bowl shaped like a kidney bean), as well as some nausea medicine. Turning your head ensures that you won't aspirate, or breathe in, your vomit.

I've found that many women get a bit queasy with the rapid onset of spinal anesthesia. Your body is undergoing a lot of changes, which can make you feel pretty weird for a few minutes. The nausea may also be due to low blood pressure. To get nauseous is one thing; throwing up is another. No one likes throwing up, but when you're having a cesarean, it can actually be dangerous. If you vomit and aspirate when getting general anesthesia, it can cause pneumonia. If the vomit is acidic, it can lead to Mendelssohn's syndrome, which is sometimes fatal. If you had significant nausea and/or vomiting during a prior cesarean, let your anesthesiologist know.

Because nausea and vomiting are so common during cesarean deliveries, many anesthesiologists give medications prophylactically. Popular medications include metoclopramide (Reglan), ondansetron (Zofran), droperidol, a small amount of a steroid called dexamethasone, and an intermediate duration acid reducer like ranitidine (Zantac) or famotidine (Pepcid).

But even with one or more of these medications, nausea can still happen. One of the extremely common pain medications, epidural or spinal morphine, can make you itchy or sometimes nauseous for twelve to twenty-four hours after the surgery. (While any narcotic can have these side effects, itching is more common when you get narcotics in your back.) Hopefully your anesthesiologist can tweak your anesthesia or medications to make the nausea manageable. If you ask the right questions and are familiar with the medications, you'll be a lot more comfortable during and after your surgery. You can help create the birth experience you want.

Take "Kate," a woman who came in for a repeat cesarean. During the birth of her first child, Kate had been in labor for thirty-six hours—and she pushed for a solid three! In the end, she'd wound up with a cesarean, which was very disappointing to her. She said she was so sleepy that she couldn't even remember the birth of her child! And after the surgery, she'd thrown up all night and the next day.

The second time around, Kate was nervous and afraid—for good reason. She'd been anxious throughout her pregnancy because her first experience was so terrible. She tearfully told me about her past experience, and how she was afraid the same thing would happen again.

I listened carefully to Kate and assured her that she would have a better experience than last time. We worked out an anesthesia plan that would keep her comfortable, reduce her chances for nausea and vomiting, and give her medications prophylactically to try and prevent any undesirable symptoms.

For the birth of her second baby, Kate was awake and alert for the surgery. She didn't throw up once and felt great the next day. She was incredibly happy and thankful when she left the hospital with her baby girl in tow.

Getting Hooked Up

Many women have told me their IV being placed was the worst part of their surgery. So that you don't have to join their ranks, here are some tips to help make it a better experience.

First, stay hydrated. Drink those clear liquids until the time you are supposed to stop drinking water. Any professional athlete will tell you that staying well-hydrated is crucial to any strenuous physical activity—including having a baby! By staying hydrated, your veins will be bigger, making them easier to find. Nobody wants to be poked ten times by a tentative nurse! Remember the baseball rule: three strikes and you're outta there. If your nurse is having a problem, there should be more experienced nurses and doctors around to help start your IV.

Your prior medical history may affect where your IV is placed. Don't hold back—go ahead and tell the nurse if you have a better spot for your IV based on previous surgeries. This information can be quite helpful to the attending staff. Just remember to be flexible if they pick a different spot. They'll put a tourniquet around your arm or forearm; repetitively squeeze your hand to pump up the veins. Then you can relax your hand.

You've already bathed with CHG at home; now be sure the person putting in your IV gives you the same courtesy. They should swab your skin with either chlorhexidine or, more commonly used among medical personnel, an isopropyl alcohol swab. He or she should also be

---

INSIDER SECRET

Peripheral IVs (the ones in your arms) should be changed every 48 hours to help prevent infection. My cousin was once in the hospital having some tests run when she realized that the same IV was left in her arm for *five days*. She developed a FUO—"Fever of Unknown Origin"—which almost certainly originated from her IV. Thanks to the FUO, she was stuck in the hospital for seven more days on a vigorous regimen of antibiotics. Don't let this happen to you.

---

wearing a glove. Make sure they place an occlusive dressing (solid barrier, typically a clear plastic) on top of the IV insertion site. This helps prevent outside bacteria from getting onto the IV puncture site and into your bloodstream.

Make sure that whenever you get medicine connected or injected through your IV line that the port (the part that goes beneath your skin) is wiped off with alcohol first. When I was taking my mother in for her chemotherapy, I remember being impressed at how good the nurse's sterile technique was with IV placement and medication administration. The oncology nurses deal with patients who have weakened immune systems and who would not be able to tolerate even a few bacteria entering their bloodstream. Unfortunately, not everyone is so meticulous. A polite way to remind your health care provider is to say, "May I get you an alcohol swab?"

Very often the IV is easiest to place in your hand—which hurts more to put in and maintain—or the wrist along the thumb side (nicknamed the "intern's vein" because it's large, straight, and easy to find). IVs can also be placed higher up in the forearm or at the crease in your arm where you bend your elbow (the antecubital vein). An IV in this location can also be a bit irritating, because every time you bend your arm it moves the IV catheter in your vein, causing pain. See the video at www.SafeBabySystem.com/IV for good ways to tape the IV so that it won't hurt you.

The size of the IV catheter matters, too. The bigger the catheter, the faster you can get fluid—a potential lifesaver in a bleeding emergency. Typically Labor & Delivery nurses will put in an 18-gauge IV. With "gauge" as the measure, the larger the number, the smaller the actual catheter (trivia buffs—gauge means how many fit in one inch—impress your nurses and doctors!). A 20-gauge IV can also be used if you really have only very small veins. Fortunately, in pregnancy, the blood flow increases and the veins typically enlarge.

The IV placement will usually hurt less if they use local anesthetic first with a teeny tiny needle (27-gauge), just to numb the skin. If your veins are small, difficult, or superficial, this may not be possible, as the local anesthetic "skin wheel" can distort the anatomy of the vein and make it harder. But it doesn't hurt to ask if they can use some local anesthetic first.

For a cesarean section, you also need to have a urine catheter placed into your bladder, called a Foley. To get to the most commonly used location where they cut into the uterus, your OB actually "takes down" or removes the bladder, which is normally adherent to the anterior surface (the way in!) of the uterus. If the doctors operate on you with a full or partially distended bladder, the likelihood of surgically cutting or "nicking" the bladder goes way up. So make sure the Foley catheter is draining your bladder well (urine flowing into reservoir bag) after insertion and before they start surgery. The soft Foley tube can twist or kink, causing obstruction and preventing good drainage.

By the way: make sure to ask that they do the Foley AFTER you get the anesthesia so that you don't feel it. Many women do get the Foley awake and non-anesthetized, but why go through the pain and discomfort if you don't have to? You'll thank me for this tip, as will your body. It's been through enough!

After they start your IV, you will need to get 1 liter of crystalloid—basically salt water. Enjoy it: it's your breakfast, lunch, or dinner. Aside from making you feel better, this extra boost of hydration is important before you get your anesthetic. The spinal and epidural anesthetics cause not only numbness, but also dilate your blood vessels and can drop your blood pressure.

Many women feel a bit weird or even nauseous right after the regional (spinal or epidural) anesthesia for a C-section, mostly due to changes in your cardiovascular system. The anesthetics cause vasodilation of your blood vessels, and if your "tank" is less than full, the blood return to the heart is lower, and the volume your heart can pump decreases. That's why you feel woozy. And if you're woozy, it means your baby is getting less blood flow, too. So make sure you get your liter of fluid BEFORE going to the OR. You'll feel better for it, as will your baby.

* * *

They're finally wheeling you out of pre-op and into the OR for your cesarean. You're hydrated, you're calm, and you're prepared. Now let's bring your baby into the world!

Things To Keep In Mind

- Preparing properly for your trip to the hospital to give birth is extremely important.

- Leave the jewelry home and keep your makeup light.

- Cleanse yourself thoroughly before leaving for the hospital. consider washing with CHG on your skin. Ideally, shave or wax the day before your C-section.

- Keep a copy of your personal medical history with you the last trimester, including medication names and doses as well as any surgeries you have had.

- Be sure to tell your nurse and anesthesiologist about ALL your allergies, not just about any allergies to medicines. Some food allergies cross react with medications!

- Know your medicines and keep a complete list with you at all times.

- If you're having a repeat cesarean section, an ultrasound is especially important for the OB to know the location of the placenta.

- Know and follow the rules your hospital suggests regarding eating and drinking the day of the C-section.

- Don't hold back—go ahead and tell the nurse if you have a better spot for your IV based on previous surgeries.

- Make sure to ask that they do the Foley AFTER you get the anesthesia so that you don't feel it.

Go to www.SafeBabySystem.com/bonus for additional information.

REFERENCES

[i] Dumas AM. Eur J Obstet Gynecol Reproduct BIol 2009:147:139-143. Maternal infection rates after cesarean delivery by Pfannenstiel or Joel-Cohen incision: a multicenter surveillance study.

[ii] Trenev N. Probiotics: Nature's Internal Healers, Avery Publishing Garden City 1998.p57.

[iii] American Society of Anesthesiologists, "What you should know about herbal and dietary supplement use and anesthesia." http://www.asahq.org/patientEducation/herb Patient.pdf.

[iv] Silver RM. Obstet Gynecol 2006:107:1226-32. Maternal morbidity associated with multiple repeat cesarean deliveries.

[v] Practice Guidelines for preoperative fasting and use of pharmacologic agents to reduce the risk of pulmonary aspiration: application to healthy patients undergoing elective procedures. Anesthesiology 1999:90:896-905.

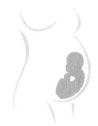

Chapter 6

Intra-Op: Surviving Your Stitch in Time

Welcome to the Operating Room—my home away from home. Many women consider the OR a daunting place, but it doesn't have to be. I want to make sure your stay in the OR is as comfortable as can be.

In this chapter, we will walk through everything that is going to go on during your cesarean so that nothing is strange or unexpected. We'll begin from when you first enter the OR and end with the moment you're holding your healthy newborn in your arms. Because you'll be familiar with the entire process, you'll quiet the fears and feel the stress and anxiety melt away as you enjoy the beautiful birth of your child.

Through the Doors

Your trip to the operating room won't always be a journey by gurney; you may very well walk into the OR. You'll be wearing a hospital gown, so make sure your back is covered, as those silly gowns expose your posterior. To keep your derriere safely concealed, either double up on gowns—one facing forward, one facing backwards—or use a blanket to wrap yourself up. Just make sure the blanket is long enough to cover your backside!

If you're slated for a walk-in trip, you'll be stepping up onto the OR table and will probably use a step stool to do so. Use this opportunity to remove your extra layers as the anesthesiologist will almost certainly need to get to your back.

If you are going from labor to cesarean, they will be rolling you into the OR on your bed. If you already have an epidural, you will probably be a bit numb and it may be difficult to move yourself to the OR table. Here is an insider's trick: if your legs are a bit heavy, have someone bring your feet over the OR table and hold them down. Then you can use your arms to lift your body and swing your butt across. If your legs feel so heavy that even this maneuver seems an impossible feat, you may be placed on a roller-type board to help pull you onto the operating table.

On the Table

Before your anesthesia or the start of surgery, new regulations require the doctors to call a "time out" before starting any procedure. They state your name, allergies, antibiotics, special equipment, and medications. Although this was considered a bit of a nuisance until everyone got used to it, I think it's a great way to make sure everyone is on the same page.

Once that's been established and you are on the OR table, monitors will be applied. The standard monitors include ECG, BP, and pulse oximeter. Let's walk through each one.

The ECG monitors the electrical conduction of your heart, as seen on popular TV shows like *ER*. There should be a tracing, accompanied by a slow and steady beeping sound. When the Bovie is being used, the electric current interferes with the ECG and you get a fuzzy or irregular tracing. Don't worry—this will stop as soon as they stop using the Bovie, and your heart rate as shown on the monitor will return to normal (between 60 and 120 beats per minute).

There are several other events that can affect the quality of the ECG tracing, such as shivering, shaking, or electrical interference. Sometimes it's hard to get an accurate tracing if the ECG pads are not sticky or property placed, or if the ECG wire is loose or broken. The alarm will go off or the heart rate number will be too high or low. Knowing to look out for these things will save you time and stress wondering what's wrong when you're in the OR.

Then there's the automated blood pressure machine, called a NIBP: Non-Invasive Blood Pressure, that will take your blood pressure. When I started training in anesthesiology, we had to take the blood pressure manually throughout the entire cesarean. Things are much easier now. However, the NIBP can still be somewhat fickle. And be warned: the first time it inflates, it might hurt a little because the cuff pumps up so high.

The machine measures the blood pressure by detecting the vibrations of the artery from the cuff, feeding those vibrations into the machine and as the cuff slowly deflates. Since the machine reads the vibrations, any movement by your arm throws off the reading. It's sensitive to both big movements, like moving your arm to scratch your nose, but is also attuned to smaller movements, like shaking or shivering. When you feel the cuff starting to inflate, you can help it to finish faster and be more accurate if you hold your arm straight and still. Sometimes you can't avoid shivering when you are cold, but try your best. Unfortunately shivering occurs quite commonly.

Although difficulty getting the blood pressure machine to read properly is 99 percent due to mechanical/shaking problems, it can also be from very low blood pressure. Errors occur when staff fuss with the machine first, then look at the patient second. This is when your labor partner is key to your safety! He or she should be looking out for you, including things like your blood pressure. If the NIBP isn't reading properly, have your partner call for help.

Once it's clear that you are okay, your nurse can try moving the cuff to another place, like your leg. Since you're already numb there, your leg won't shake. And if all else fails, there's always the old-fashioned way: taking your blood pressure manually or even just by feeling your pulse ('palp' pressure).

INSIDER SECRET

INSIDER SECRET

Warning Signs of Low Blood Pressure:

- Mentally not as alert
- Pallor (looks drained in face)
- Sweaty
- Feeling Weird (e.g. tunnel vision)
- Light headed
- Machine not able to take Blood pressure

Do NOT waste time letting someone futz forever with the blood pressure machine! Get a nurse or doctor to the bedside right away!

This tip could save someone's life.

The next piece of equipment you'll see on the OR table is the pulse oximeter—one of the best inventions in the last thirty years. The pulse oximeter puts two special frequencies of light through the capillaries in your nail bed to measure the oxygen saturation. Oxygen saturation is the percent of hemoglobin (the stuff carrying oxygen around the body) in your red blood cells that has oxygen attached to it. Prior to the availability and standard use of pulse oximeters, we had to look at a patient's skin color and the color of their blood to guesstimate whether they had enough oxygen.

Modern technological improvements have ushered in a new era of certainty; these days safety tests are far more easy and reliable. The pulse oximeter allows your Anesthesiologist to continuously monitor your oxygen saturation to catch a trend or problem before it continues long enough to cause damage to you or your baby. Most machines have a certain tone to the saturation, so you get an auditory confirmation—the tone of the beep lowers as the oxygen saturation drops. The better you know these tones, the more calm you'll feel on the day of your C-section. For additional information see www.SafeBabySystem.com.

Getting Cozy

Generally, the OR is maintained at a cold level—low 60s °F, allegedly to keep the bacterial count down. In truth, it may have more to do with keeping the people who are "gowned" up in surgical garb from sweating.

No one wants a sweaty surgeon. Or, for that matter, a sweaty surgical assistant, scrub tech, or scrub nurse.

However, recent studies show the importance of YOU being warm. Many body processes, including the ability to fight infection, are dependent on having a normal body temperature.[i] Hypothermia (low body temperature) not only increases infections at the site of surgery; it also increases the demands on your heart. Warming your IV fluids can help keep you warmer, meaning you'll shiver less and get out of the recovery room faster.[ii] Even national organizations such as the AHRQ (The Agency for Healthcare Research and Quality) have started to require patients undergoing larger surgical procedures like colon resections to end the surgery warm. Sadly, requirements for cesarean sections are slow to catch up to the trend.

Fortunately, you can make a difference when it comes to temperature management. Ask for the OR temperature to be warmed up *before* you get there. If the room is warm, everything you touch is warm—your bed, IV fluid, BP cuff, everything. Then, after your anesthesia, after your prep, and after you are draped, the temperature can be turned down, so as to keep the sweating down to a minimum. This is easy to request, doesn't cost anyone any extra time or energy, and is definitely good for you. Ask your OB or your anesthesiologist.

> **INSIDER SECRET**
>
> On the night shift at a Midwestern hospital, a nurse shared with me some of his "clinical pearls." He told me that when he had a patient who was cold, he placed one of the plastic bags of IV fluids into the microwave to heat it up. That way, he said, he could warm the patient. I was aghast. A nurse should NEVER put IV fluids in a microwave! Since you can't control the temperature, the plastic might decay if too hot or lose sterility, and you can get thermal burn from the fluid itself if it enters your vein at too hot a temperature. Micro-waving is NOT the answer. In search of trying to help, people do the darndest things. So congrats on learning what goes on, the right things to do, and the right questions to ask!

Other tips for staying warm include having your IV fluid run through a fluid warmer (may not be needed if the room is reasonably warm at the get-to). There are different types of fluid warmers. One of the most common is HotLine, which is very good for warming fluids to body temperature. However, if the fluid is dripping in slowly, it will lose some heat before it even gets to you. For very fast fluid administration, there are pressurized fluid warmers, like the Level 1. You can transfuse a unit of blood in about 5 minutes through a good IV with one of these. A rapid transfuser can be a life-saver in a pinch. Make sure the hospital has at least one of these in Labor & Delivery.

You can also request that your fluids be placed in a heated cabinet before they're given to you. These are used in most ORs for blankets, irrigation fluids, and IV fluids. Just make sure the fluid isn't over-warm —if your IV site feels hot, speak up and have them turn it off.

Here's a simple, homey trick: bring a pair of those warm fuzzy socks and wear them. I had a patient just the other day who wore very large, very soft fluffy socks. She said they helped keep her warm, and she was right—she didn't shiver once during the spinal or after we prepped and draped her. If you don't mind that they might get dirty, most doctors and nurses will allow you to keep your socks on during a cesarean. And they look cute, too.

Shivering during the surgery is fairly common, even with all these tricks. At least half the women I've seen have a cesarean delivery shiver at some point. This is partly due to being half naked in a typically cold environment, partly due to the way the heat within your body shifts under regional anesthesia, and partly hormonal (many women shiver, even with vaginal deliveries and no anesthesia). Shivering or jaw-shaking can lead to sore muscles in your neck after delivery. Ask for a warm blanket, or better yet, a warming blanket or a hot air blower. A good old-fashioned neck rub can work wonders, too.

Many women experience neck pain during a cesarean section. Part of that is due to anxiety—they've been holding a lot of tension in their necks. Make sure that your pillow is comfortable for you when you are lying down. A trick I often use is to roll the pillow so there is more neck support than if the pillow is just lying flat.

You may also experience shoulder pain during and after surgery. Generally for a cesarean, your arms are not tied down, and you are free to move them—as long as you move them laterally (out to the side, your face, or your upper chest). Just remember not to scratch your belly—the surgeon does not want your inadvertent help during surgery! Also, check that your arms are not swung up at too great an angle (you know your own body and how far you can raise your arms). If need be, you can ask to have your arms across your chest to minimize aching shoulders.

Sometimes, though, shoulder pain is actually "referred pain" from something—either air or blood—under the diaphragm. During the cesarean, blood or air can travel up the abdominal cavity between the liver and the diaphragm. Your body's nerves tell your brain it hurts, but you feel it in the shoulder! There's not much you can do about referred pain; just know that it won't last forever. For now, cuddle up under your blanket and think cozy thoughts.

Now that you're all warm and toasty, let's talk about mood music. Most ORs come fully equipped for music. What a great opportunity to play some tunes you love! Make this your best birthing experience ever—bring your own iPod or MP3 player. You might even create a special birthing playlist that you will remember forever. If you default to the radio, you'll be at the whim of the DJ, and you might not want your baby being born to heavy metal rock.

Just remember: the music volume must be soft enough so everyone can hear each other speak and, more importantly, so the doctors and nurses can hear the monitors that are helping to guard your life (e.g., ECG, pulse oximeter). If volume is an issue, you can always bring your own music with your own set of headphones. Many couples do. Some women don't like listening to the 'shop talk' going on between the surgeons. You might even choose to listen to hypnosis tapes about being relaxed and healthy throughout your cesarean.

Different hospitals have different policies about how many people, if any, can come in during your C-section. If your hospital allows guest(s) in the OR, please remind yours to stay seated. If they get up and move around, it gets in everybody's way. The doctors will let you know when the baby is actually coming out so that your guests can stand and watch from the seated area. Abiding by these instructions will be a big help to everyone involved!

Now let's talk about media. And I don't mean the paparazzi—I mean the media you're going to create!

Most hospitals have policies about not videotaping procedures. There's an obvious concern over the medicolegal aspects of surgery, as the presence of a videocamera affects *all* the nurses and doctors, especially in Labor & Delivery. Sometimes proud dads or friends try to video the anesthesia, the monitors, the surgery—everything. While the desire to document this important day is totally understandable, your documentary filmmaker instinct does not generate warm and fuzzy feelings in any of your health care providers. Sad but true: the emotional response to video in the OR is usually a negative one. You don't really want to distract or upset your providers, even if they don't show their agitation outright.

Think of it this way: how would you feel if someone came to your place of work and started filming everything you do? When your health care providers don't have to worry about being filmed, it frees them up to do what they really like to do: take care of you, the patient. The good news is that in most hospitals, you are more than welcome to have someone video the baby once he or she has made it out of your uterus and into the wide world beyond. And the *really* good news is that you can take as many still photographs as you want!

Taking pictures of your new baby is one of the greatest joys in life. I suggest bringing a couple of cameras, a video and a still. Some of the newer electronic ones (and even the latest iPhone) do both video and still photos, although the quality is not always so professional. Just be aware that it's sometimes difficult for a dad or partner to be fully present and enjoy the moment when he's also playing photographer and videographer . . . and still trying to help his wife. Don't be afraid to ask for help—the nurses and anesthesiologists are well-versed in OR Photography 101 and will be happy to snap some shots.

I routinely offer to help take pictures of the baby, the family, and especially dad cutting the umbilical cord. I remember one couple that came in unexpectedly to the hospital and were rushed in the OR for a cesarean section. They had no camera and expressed regret that they would never have pictures of the birth. While a colleague watched mom for me, I ran out and bought a disposable camera in the gift shop, came back, and took pictures for them. The reward was all mine—to see their smiling faces and know that they would start off their new family with the pictures they always wanted.

I frequently see men in the labor room pulling out a new camera and playing with it. Most of the time they can get it to work, but sometimes a part is missing, like the right plug to charge it. If you are going to get a new camera, please check it out beforehand so that you're up to speed on delivery day. And be sure to pack extra batteries and chargers, too.

This brings me to the subject of your husband or partner and their role in the OR. Your labor partner can be a great source of comfort during your cesarean section. They can also be a great source of support, emotionally, and physically. So many moms are anxious, but with someone there holding their hand, they're able to make it through and are flooded with relief when the baby arrives.

Your birthing partner is also your advocate. If you feel ill and especially if you have a change in mental alertness, it's their job to help bring it to the attention of the doctors. Your partner should learn about the monitors in the operation room—they need to be watching the main OR monitor, the ECG, and the pulse oximeter for oxygen saturation levels. If something's not right, it's their job to sound the alarm. Your partner is your right-hand man (or woman) during your time in the OR . . . and don't let them forget it.

Got Anesthesia?

Now it's finally time to get anesthesia. Many women fear this part of the process. In fact for some moms-to-be, this is the *most* fearsome aspect of having a baby. I'm here to put your mind at ease, quieting the fears of pregnancy by guiding you through it, one step at a time. It is better to learn about this beforehand, as when emotions are high or you are in pain, it is difficult to listen or even follow instructions. You will be better prepared to help make the anesthesia placement easier, faster, and less painful, as well as reduce the chance for complications.

Let's begin by defining our terms. There are three types of anesthesia: spinal (a single injection of local anesthetic), epidural (regional anesthesia injected through a catheter into the epidural space), and general (inducing a state of complete unconsciousness). Spinal anesthesia puts local anesthetic and typically some narcotic directly into the spinal fluid (CSF). It has the advantage of being fast onset and very reliable, and it makes you extremely numb. Epidural anesthesia puts medication via a tiny tube just outside the dura, or the tough sack containing the spinal cord, spinal fluid, and nerves. The medication has to spread up, down, right and left, in order to numb up each nerve root as it exits your back. The advantages of epidural anesthesia can be slower onset, generally faster wearing off, and you can even get more medication through the catheter if the surgery goes longer than expected. If you already have an epidural for labor pain relief, you only need more medication injected via the epidural catheter to make you numb enough for surgery. Both spinal and epidural are placed within the spinal canal in your back. Neither involves injecting anything into your spinal cord! A common misconception. Now you can learn how to help make getting the anesthesia easier. We'll discuss spinal and epidural anesthesia first.

Positioning:

Most nurses and doctors underestimate the importance of proper positioning, but it's extremely important for regional (spinal or epidural) anesthesia. I'm going to share with you some tips on how to make it a lot easier for your anesthesiologist—ways that you can help to create a larger, more open target and pathway for this important procedure, thus making it easier and safer for you.

Whether you are sitting or lying down on your side will be determined by your anesthesiologist or nurse anesthetist. The decision is usually based on whichever position they are more comfortable and confident with. Just to make sure all our bases are covered, I'm going to give you tips for both.

More women tend to get into optimal position sitting rather than lying down. When you sit on the bed, whether it's an OR table or a labor bed, rather than sitting in the middle with your legs hanging down, scoot all the way back. The problem with the middle of the bed is that people tend to sink, and when they sink, it increases the chances that their body is tilted or twisted. Hospital beds and tables are built to maneuver and change positions, so there are breaks in the support structure and cut-outs for various positions. Even if you're just near one of those breaks, you tend to have your pelvis tilted in that direction. So do your anesthesiologist a favor and scoot all the way back.

It may feel funny as your legs are probably straighter in front of you than normal, but it's only for a few minutes. Now, with your pelvis firmly rooted on stable ground, just relax. (Easier said than done, I know!) That's the second most important positioning maneuver: simply to relax. Forget everything you were taught in manners class—now's the time when you *want* to slouch! If you are tense, you tense up everywhere and tighten the muscles in your back, clamping down on the space in your back where the anesthesiologist wants to go. If you think, "Slouch," then you can't help but relax, thereby releasing the tension in those back muscles.

If you are going to be on your side (in the lateral position) for your anesthesia, follow the same rules as above. You still want to be all the way on the edge of the bed closest to your anesthesiologist. Many L&D nurses prefer the lateral position because it is easier for them to monitor the baby during placement of the anesthesia. The key to rounding your lower back out in the lateral position is your pelvis. Tilt your pelvis forward. Here's another insider's secret—bring your knees up to your chest. This automatically rounds the lower part of your back out, opening up the spaces between your vertebrae. It really is that easy!

After your skin is cleaned with the antiseptic, a sterile drape (paper or plastic) will be placed over your back. The drape helps extend the sterile work area and prevent contamination by bacteria or other unwanted stuff like linen fluff.

Here's how it works: first your skin is numbed up with local anesthetic via a tiny (should be 27-gauge, 25-gauge max) needle. You'll feel a pinch and a slight burning before it goes numb. Then, many doctors (I certainly do!) numb up the deeper part of the skin with a somewhat larger, longer needle. After that you should just feel pressure, albeit in a weird spot where you're not used to getting injections.

If you feel pain, speak up. If you feel the needle on one side, say so! You are an important part of the geography conversation . . . actually, the most important part. If the needle is off to one side, then the deeper it goes, the more "off sides" the tip becomes. Since the epidural veins and nerve roots are actually lateral and more prone to get traumatized if the needle goes there, it's important that you say something if things feel off kilter. You're not being a nuisance; you're being a huge help! You will actually help to make it less painful and decrease chance of paresthesias (nerve twinges, or electric shock sensation).

The spinal anesthetic kicks in quickly and densely. You will feel the warmth spreading from your buttocks or legs almost immediately. Within a few minutes, the sensation will come up to your mid-chest. You want to get a T4 level—meaning you are numb up to your Thoracic 4th vertebrae—easier to identify as your mid-chest or nipple line. Even though the incision is low on your abdomen, the peritoneum (inner lining of the abdominal cavity) goes all the way up to and behind your liver and spleen. So to be comfortable during a cesarean, you need to numb up to the T4 sensory level.

Epidural anesthesia works the same way; it just takes a few minutes longer. And though it takes longer at the beginning, things do speed up at the end; a side benefit of epidural

INSIDER SECRET

There is also something called a CSE (combined spinal epidural), one of the newer techniques available. A CSE can speed the onset of pain relief, sometimes within just a few minutes. When the initial epidural needle is in the right spot, a smaller "spinal" needle is inserted to deliver medicine directly into the spinal fluid. Some doctors swear by it, but in my experience, the potential for additional risks and side effects—studies are as of yet inconclusive, but possible risks include an increase in temporary FHR abnormalities and nerve damage—far outweigh the benefits.

anesthesia for cesarean delivery is that it usually wears off faster. That means you can get out of the recovery room (or PACU—post anesthesia care unit) about an hour faster. With an epidural, you may feel a bit more of the pressure and pulling, as it is on average not quite as dense as with spinal anesthesia. Remember that the epidural medication has to spread up and down, left and right, numbing up each nerve root as it is coming out of your back. In other words: it's got more work to do.

OR Table & supine positioning:

The tables in the OR are intentionally very narrow. After all, the OR is a business district, not a hotel room. The bed is narrow so that everyone can get in close to your body—the principle site of interest. What most women don't know is that a mere two inches can make a huge difference, especially for your back and neck. This is particularly true with spinal anesthesia—because it makes you numb very quickly, you want to make sure when you first lie down on the table that you are centered in the bed. Start by centering your hips. Then make sure your shoulders are aligned evenly with your hips, in neutral position.

If your shoulders are even slightly misaligned, you will have torque on your spine. Normally, you might be able to sustain that for a few minutes before you get uncomfortable and subconsciously shifted your position. However, when you are under anesthesia—whether numb from regional anesthesia or asleep from general anesthesia—you won't feel the discomfort, and you certainly won't be able to shift into a more natural position. Thus you stand a decent chance of having some musculoskeletal aches or even exacerbation of a preexisting back problem. Make sure you do a survey of your body and positioning before you are prepped and draped – you are helping to reduce or prevent back pain after your cesarean.

Part of positioning for a cesarean section involves LUD, or left uterine displacement. Many doctors and nurses place a sandbag or something similar under your right hip to displace and tilt your pelvis 15-30 degrees to the left. Utilizing LUD shifts the weight of the uterus and baby off the low-pressure inferior vena cava (large vein), moving it onto the spine and high-pressure aorta (large artery). When you are totally flat on your back, the pressure from the weight of the baby compresses the inferior vena cava, thereby reducing blood return to the heart. Without adequate blood flow returning to your heart, your heart pumps less blood around the body, resulting in a drop in maternal blood pressure and a decreased blood supply to the baby.

Personally, I just tilt the whole OR table to the left side. That avoids twisting the pelvis relative to the spine, resulting in fewer complaints of back pain. Your anesthesiologist may have a different technique. Either way, just make sure you are tilted a bit to the left, at least until your baby is born.

Pillow Talk

If you have back pain or tend to get back twinges, another helpful tip – make sure they put a small pillow under your knees. A pillow under your knees will help to straighten out the lumbar spine, helping to reduce back pain later. Some surgeons don't like a big pillow, as the knees will be pushed too high up and can sometimes get in the way. Speaking of pillow talk—use pillows to cushion the bony parts of your legs—between the knees and between your legs and the bedrail during labor or after surgery. Another tip from Safe Baby System Chapter 11— during labor be sure to rest your legs between pushes. Too often, helpful staff (and over-eager husbands) push the legs too far back, flexing your hips and pushing your knees towards your chest. This can strain and tear the muscles and nerves. In certain cases where the labor team has been a little too over-zealous, I've seen women who could barely walk the next day!

Once you're in position, either sitting up or lying down, your back will be scrubbed with an antiseptic. The standard solution was tradition-ally an iodine-based antiseptic called povidine/iodine (Betadyne). The national recommendation has changed to using another antiseptic combination on the skin that immediately kills the bacteria but with a prolonged effect: alcohol with chlorhexidine. Alcohol is still the best agent for immediate disinfection, and the chlorhexidine sticks to the skin and provides prolonged antibacterial effect. It's the new golden child in antiseptics. Just make sure they give it enough time (typically 2 minutes) for the alcohol to totally evaporate. Because alcohol is flammable, if you don't wait for it to dry before using electrocautery, you can cause a fire.

Testing, testing…is your anesthesia ok?

For both spinal and epidural anesthesia, your anesthesiologist will perform several simple tests before the cesarean begins. Typically you will be checked to see how high the spinal or epidural block has become, oftentimes with a cold sensation test (e.g., alcohol swipe) or with a pinprick. Don't worry—the surgeon will check to make sure you are very numb before they attempt skin incision (the first cut through the skin). Most often, the OB checks with a sharp-toothed forceps clamp called an Allis clamp. The surgeon will also check that you are numb using an Allis clamp before making the first incision on your skin. Take it from me: the clamp test is quite effective!

Once in a while, there might still be some discomfort right at the skin incision, even though you are pretty numb. If this happens, the surgeon can either wait for the epidural medicine to finish kicking in, or inject a little local anesthetic right along the superficial skin incision site. The nerve fibers that end in the midline are the last to get numb during an epidural because they are the deepest within that nerve bundle. In a dire life and death emergency where the baby's life is at risk, the surgeon can always numb up each layer with a local anesthetic before cutting to get the baby out.[iii] Often, the surgeon is in a rush when this is needed and the deeper layers aren't completely numb. Of course most mothers are more than willing to endure a little pain for a live baby in a dire emergency. One more reason why choosing a hospital with 24/7 dedicated OB anesthesia staffing pays off.

General Anesthesia:

Now let's talk about general anesthesia. If you are receiving a general anesthetic, then either regional anesthetic is relatively contraindicated (blood not clotting well, infection over your back, low blood volume), or there is no time to do a spinal or epidural (baby or mom's life is at imminent risk). General anesthesia is relatively safe, but not as safe as regional. The data from a 1998 study showed that maternal death by anesthesia was sixteen times higher with general than with regional.[iv] New data recently presented shows this relative risk of death by anesthesia has improved to about three times higher for general compared to regional. Fortunately, the absolute risk of death by anesthesia is remarkably small: only one out of 500,000, thanks to advances by Anesthesiologists in the last 20+ years.[v]

Here's all you need to remember for general anesthesia: take a deep breath. And I mean that literally—you need to replace the room air (79 percent nitrogen) in your lungs with 100 percent oxygen. That way, in the short period of time you aren't breathing during the intubation (placing of the breathing tube), you'll have plenty of oxygen in your lungs as a kind of "reserve tank" in case of difficulty or delay.

Keep taking deep breaths—as deeply as you can—as you drift off to sleep. This will keep you partly breathing and exchanging oxygen for longer as you start down the road to total unconsciousness. I've seen this simple trick make the difference from staying 100 percent saturated with oxygen and having your oxygen level start to drop off. This is better for you, the baby, and my coronaries, too!

Typically you will not be "put out" until the OB is nearly ready. The longer you, the mom, are under general anesthesia, the more the general anesthesia has time to transfer to the baby, making the baby a little sleepy when he or she comes out. By waiting until the OB is ready to perform the surgery, your baby receives less drugs.

Once you're numb and properly situated and prepped on the OR table, they're going to put the drapes up. Great! That means they're about to start. If you are claustrophobic, make sure to tell your anesthesiologist so they can try to push the drape back a bit from your face. Once the drapes are up, they'll bring your spouse or labor partner into the OR.

Lights, Camera, CUT!

So you're good and numb and the OB has made the first incision. Now what can you expect?

After getting through the layers of skin and muscle, the abdominal cavity is opened up. Occasionally some women are comfortable during the first part of the surgery, but feel some discomfort when the abdominal cavity is opened. To ensure that this doesn't happen, the anesthesiologist needs to raise the level of the anesthesia all the way up to your mid chest to make sure the whole inner lining of the abdominal cavity, the peritoneum, is numb. Remember—speak up and tell your anesthesiologist or nurse anesthetist if you feel any pain or discomfort.

The next step involves taking the bladder down off the uterus. The bladder is normally attached to the anterior surface of the uterus (toward your front side), and gets pulled up as the uterus grows during pregnancy. During a cesarean, the bladder is carefully separated from the uterus and pulled down. Then a metal bladder blade is inserted to protect the bladder and help expose the uterus. Very infrequently, the bladder is nicked during this procedure, which would necessitate repair at the end of surgery. In case of a major tear, you might need a urine catheter (Foley) to be left in place for a while until the bladder heals and forms a complete seal again. A urogynecologist or urologist may be called in to ensure a proper repair.

Once the bladder is moved, your baby is about to be born! You'll normally hear the surgeon ask the scrub tech for "knife, bandage-scissors" as they make the uterine incision. That signals that birth is imminent, as they will then use the scissors to cut the uterus open. The uterine incision to delivery time should be less than 3 minutes.

If it takes longer, it means they are having a hard time getting the baby out. Once the uterus is opened, the baby may not be getting his or her full supply of blood and thus oxygen. At this point, the surgeon may ask for a vacuum to help pull the baby's head up and out. Nothing to worry about just yet—just follow how long it takes to get the baby out and how many attempts are made. More than 3 minutes or a couple of attempts indicates that the OB is having trouble getting the head out, typically from a head that was wedged into the birth canal.

Once the baby's head (or butt, if in breech position) is out of the uterus, the assistant surgeon presses hard on your abdomen to help the baby come out of the uterine incision. A combination of pushing on your upper belly and pulling on the baby's head and neck provide the power to take the baby out. Since you are numb up to your chest, you'll feel the pressure in your chest and may have some difficulty breathing. That's normal—after all, there's a lot of pressure on your upper stomach area. I'd have trouble breathing if someone was pushing on my chest, too!

The baby is officially born when the entire body is outside of you. The OB usually suctions the mouth with a bulb syringe or DeLee soft suction trap. The umbilical cord is clamped and cut, and the OB passes the baby out of the surgical field and to the nurse.

Your baby is then placed in the infant warmer/bassinet. The infant warmer should be PRE-heated so the baby goes directly into a warm environment. Being small and all wet, the baby can lose heat rapidly. A drop in body temperature may lead to persistent fetal circulation and the baby may even turn blue. If all is as it should be, the warmer will be at just the right temperature and your baby will be a nice rosy shade of pink.

One of the first steps the nurse will take is to dry your baby off with a towel. Then, if the baby is not already pink and crying, she will be stimulated by rubbing her back or flicking the soles of her feet. Usually this light stimulus is enough to stimulate the baby to take a deep breath and cry.

Now comes the delivery of the afterbirth, or placenta. Your labor partner cannot cut the umbilical cord during a cesarean section like during a vaginal delivery. They'd have to be scrubbed into the surgical field! But your partner in the OR can trim the umbilical cord soon after the birth, when the baby is stable in the infant warmer. The nurse will hold the umbilical cord up so that he or she can cut between the umbilical cord clamp and a surgical clamp. Don't worry—there are no pain nerves in the umbilical cord, so your baby feels no pain. The umbilical cord is kind of squishy, so all your partner need do is make one swift, firm cut with the scissors, or two cuts if needed.

INSIDER SECRET

If these general initial steps don't help, your baby may need some neonatal resuscitation. The nurses are usually the ones who do this, although this varies from place to place. In larger hospitals, there may always be pediatrics residents around who come in to help, or in some smaller hospitals, the respiratory therapist. A neonatologist may be required when things are not going well or if the baby is experiencing more serious problems.

The hospital collects a little cord blood for testing on the baby's behalf, like to ascertain blood type. In addition, they do testing for some genetic diseases, such as PKU, a disorder that can lead to mental retardation, brain damage, and seizures if not treated. However, if PKU is detected at birth, it can lead to proper control and normal development, often causing little or no side effects.

These days, more and more parents are choosing to do umbilical cord blood banking, also called stem cell collection. You've no doubt heard of the controversy over stem cell research. But there's no controversy here. You can choose to save the stem cells—the original cells that can form any type of cell in your body—for possible later usage. The more stem cells you retrieve, the more blood you've collected, and the better it is for later use.

> **INSIDER SECRET**
>
> Oxytocin is used during a Cesarean. If you are collecting cord blood, the oxytocin should be started immediately after cord clamping. Because oxytocin helps the uterus to contract, starting it early will help the uterus to contact, squeezing the placenta, and increasing the collection of cold blood. And mom will lose less blood, too!

The umbilical cord blood is collected sterilely and sent to the company you personally contract with, where they spin the blood in a special way to collect the stem cells. After spinning and extracting the stem cells, they are deep frozen and placed in storage. The situations those stem cells can be used for are currently very limited, but if your child needed the kind of radiation and/or chemotherapy that requires stem cell/bone marrow transplant, the stem cells could be used.

I currently know one remarkable twelve-year-old battling leukemia who was told three different times over the course of one year that she only had a few weeks to live. She received her stem cell/bone marrow transplant one month ago, and today she is 100 percent in remission. Tell *that* to the doctors who told her to go home and stop fighting!

Miracle stories like this are sure to abound in the years to come. What all will they be able to do with stem cells in the future? Grow you a new liver? A new eye? Stem cells injected into brain-damaged individuals have had some reports of new growth and repairing the brain. As scientists learn to control the growth and differentiation of stem cells, the possibilities seem limitless. There are also reports of being able to harvest some cells from your skin as an adult and make them just as useful as stem cells. The answers to these questions, and many others, await.

> **INSIDER SECRET**
>
> If you become uncomfortable when they exteriorize the uterus, the anesthesia level may not be high or dense enough. Tell your anesthesiologist that it hurts. Most women feel this as discomfort in the chest since your lower parts are numb. If more medicine doesn't help and you are in a lot of discomfort, ask if they can sew the uterus inside of you. When a body part is pulled outside of the body, it creates a lot of pulling and tugging that is transmitted all the way up the abdominal cavity into your chest. If your OB can stitch your uterus up inside of you instead, you'll require less anesthesia and experience less visceral (organ) pain.

Sewing You Up Again

After the umbilical cord is collected, the placenta is removed from the uterus. During a vaginal delivery, the placenta delivers spontaneously a few minutes after the birth (hence the term "afterbirth"). And if you tug on the umbilical cord to pull the placenta out prematurely, the cord can snap, increasing bleeding. However, during a cesarean, the uterus is open and the placenta is just sitting there. So most OBs manually extract the placenta at little risk to you.

The vast majority of OBs exteriorize the uterus, or pull it out of the abdomen, to sew it back up. That's right—the uterus is actually pulled out of the pelvis and abdomen and yanked out on top of your skin right after delivery of the baby and the placenta. In the old days, the OB would sew the uterus back together when it was inside you, but having the uterus on the outside makes it a little easier to sew back together. However, having the uterus sewn back up externally can often lead to more pain for you during the first twenty-four hours.[vi]

After the uterus is fully repaired, it is pushed back into the abdomen. When the uterus was pulled out, it was soft. When it is put back inside, it is firm, and can be harder to push back in through a small incision. It's normal to feel a little discomfort at this point of the surgery.

The OB's next step is to sew up the peritoneum. The peritoneum, the inner lining of the abdomen, is repaired by being lifted up and sewn together. This step puts a lot of tugging and pulling on the peritoneum, and because of its high degree of parasympathetic nervous system innervation, you may experience some nausea, accompanied by a slight drop in blood pressure. Unfortunately, medicines don't work very well for the type of nausea instigated by your nervous system. Rest assured that it will go away in a few minutes when they've finished sewing that layer.

After the peritoneum, your OB will sew the rest of the abdominal wall—the fascia and muscles—back together. At this point, even if you were slightly uncomfortable before, you should be feeling good again. Once you are outside of the abdominal cavity, the surgical stimulation goes way down, and you need a much lower level of anesthesia to keep the pain and discomfort at bay.

> **INSIDER SECRET**
>
> Sometimes you just gotta cough. It's totally understandable. But coughing at certain points of the operation makes it really tough for the surgeon to do her job. Can you imagine sewing delicate tissue together when it is jiggling? If you're worried about coughing at an inopportune moment, ask your anesthesiologists about certain medications (e.g. narcotics) that act as cough suppressants. The strongest prescription cough syrups actually contain codeine!

Amongst the OB community, doctors vary in the types of skin closures they do. One type, nicknamed the "staple," is the fastest to close. After sewing the deepest layer to the skin, the OB takes a toothed forceps to

---

INSIDER SECRET

Some surgeons use more layers in suturing you back together while others use fewer. The "less is more" crowd says that you don't need to sew all the individual layers. The "more layers is better" advocates swear that having a tight tissue approximation helps you heal better. Certainly the fewer layers there are to sew, the faster the surgery finishes.

---

pick up the skin, pucker it up and out, and then staple the edges together. If you were to peek at this stage, you would be looking straight onto the edges of your skin. The theory goes that the skin will heal, and when they remove the staples in a few days, the scar will invert and become buried into the deeper layer of the skin so that you don't see it.

Another popular type of closure is the subcuticular closure. OBs who choose this type of closure run a suture along the very edge of the skin, back and forth, so that the skin is held very close together and tight. Some OBs spend a great deal of time doing a "plastics" closure to get the nicest, tiniest scar they can. A plastic surgery closure involves putting more sutures into the layers beneath the skin to provide more support and relieve tension on the very superficial skin layer. This allows it to heal without the occasional tugging which can pull the skin apart, resulting in a smaller scar. Of course, your basic body type and nutritional status affect how well you heal as well.

* * *

Having a cesarean can be scary, but it's always a lot scarier in your mind than in real life. I'm reminded of "Tabitha," a young woman delivering her first child several years ago. Tabitha was about as anxious as an expectant mother can get. Because she was especially terrified by the thought of any kind of surgery, she opted for natural childbirth. Since she was strong and in good health, all her doctors happily signed off on it, and everything was expected to go smoothly.

Then, something went wrong during the delivery. Tabitha needed an emergency cesarean and there wasn't much time. She was totally distraught and shaking like a leaf. She'd heard a whole slew of nightmare stories about C-sections and could only imagine the worst. Tabitha was utterly convinced that if there was an operation, she and her baby would die. It was as if all her worst fears were coming true.

As we rolled Tabitha into the OR, I told her everything would be okay. I assured her that I would be there with her during both the anesthesia and throughout her delivery, promising to keep the lines of communication open so that she never felt in the dark.

I was determined not to put Tabitha to sleep—I try not to do general anesthesia unless it's absolutely necessary, and I wanted her to witness the miracle of life. Because she was still shaking a good deal, it was imperative that she stop moving around so we could administer the spinal anesthesia. So I took her hand as the nurse helped her in position, and I talked her through every step of her spinal—just like I've done here in this book.

As I continued talking, Tabitha's fears slowly dissipated. The anesthesia was successful and she stopped shaking. The more I spoke with her about what was going on, the less afraid she felt. Because she was conscious, I was able to show her the baby being born in a mirror. She was awestruck. She continued holding my hand until after the baby was out, but she was no longer afraid.

Her baby was born beautiful and healthy, and Tabitha had overcome one of her worst fears. I can still remember the radiance of her smile as she held her firstborn child. To me, that look said, "Now I can survive anything."

On that note, let's talk about some special events that could happen during your cesarean . . . and how to survive them.

Things To Keep In Mind

Generally, the OR is maintained at a cold level—low 60s °F, allegedly to keep the bacterial count down. In truth, it may have more to do with keeping the people who are "gowned" up in surgical garb from sweating. You'll shiver less if the OR is warm. Ask.

- Bring warm, fuzzy socks to keep yourself warm during the surgery.

- Learn how to optimally position yourself for anesthesia— make it easier, faster, and less painful.

- During placement of anesthesia—speak up if you feel the needle on the side instead of in the middle. You'll reduce the pain and chance of nerve twinges.

- Learn how to lie down on the OR table correctly after the anesthesia—so you don't have back pains from having your back torqued.

- Different hospitals have different policies about how many people, if any, can come in during your C-section. If your hospital allows guest(s) in the OR, please remind yours to stay seated.

- Most hospitals have policies about not videotaping procedures.

- Sometimes it's difficult for a dad or partner to be fully present and enjoy the moment when he's also playing photographer and videographer . . . and still trying to help his wife. So enlist an OR person—a nurse or an anesthesiologist—they're used to taking those pictures!

- If you are going to get a new camera, please check it out beforehand so that you're up to speed on delivery day. And be sure to pack extra batteries and chargers, too.

- Many women experience neck or shoulder pain during a cesarean section. Rolling the pillow can make you more comfortable.

- Your birthing partner is also your advocate. If you feel ill and especially if you have a change in mental alertness, it's their job to help bring it to the attention of the doctors and nurses.

- If you are claustrophobic, make sure to tell your anesthesiologist so they can push the drape back a bit from your face.

- If you feel pain, speak up.

- General anesthesia is relatively safe, but not as safe as regional. If you have general, keep taking deep breaths— as deeply as you can—as you drift off to sleep.

- The uterine incision to delivery time should be less than 3 minutes.

- If your baby doesn't "pink up" after a minute or two, ask for the attending pediatrician or neonatologist to come and assist.

- Amongst the OB community, doctors vary in the types of skin closures they do. Discuss which one you would like.

Go to www.SafeBabySystem.com/bonus for additional information.

REFERENCES

[i] Forbes S. et al. Evidence-Based Guidelines for Prevention of Perioperative Hypothermia. J Am Coll Surg 2009:209:492-503.

[ii] Hasankhani H, et al. The Effects of Warming Intravenous Fluid on Perioperative Hemodynamic Status, Postoperative Shivering and Recovery in Orthopedic Surgery. Shiraz E-Medical Journal Vol. 5, No. 3, July 2004.

[iii] ACOG Practice Bulletin NUMBER 36, JULY 2002 Obstetric Analgesia and Anesthesia.

[iv] Hawkins JL. Anesthesiology 1997:86:277-84. Anesthesia-related deaths during obstetric delivery in the United States, 1979-1990.

[v] Hawkins JL. Anesthesiology 1997:86:277-84. Anesthesia-related deaths during obstetric delivery in the United States, 1979-1990.

[vi] Lavand'homme P. Editorial. Chronic pain after vaginal and cesarean delivery: a reality questioning our daily practice of obstetric anesthesia. Int J Obstet Anesth 2010:19:1-2.

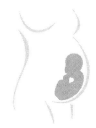

Chapter 7

Is That Supposed to Happen?

Chances are very good that your cesarean will proceed without a problem. Most do. However, because this is surgery, there are many special circumstances that can arise. Some problems are routine, while other problems are rare but life-threatening. The more knowledgeable you are about these problems, the more prepared you'll be, and the less fear you'll have if something does go wrong. In this chapter, we'll walk through all the things that could happen during your C-section, and how you can best respond to ensure that you and your baby are just fine. Don't think of them as "problems"; think of them as "events."

To begin, take a look at Figure 7.1. These are some of the most common symptoms you may experience during your cesarean. By familiarizing yourself with what they mean, you'll be less alarmed on surgery day. As President Franklin D Roosevelt said, "the only thing we have to fear is fear itself".

Look Out for the RFO!

Before they start the surgery, you will probably hear the circulating nurse and scrub tech counting the instruments, lap pads (absorbent cotton pads with a strip so they can be detected by x-ray), and needles. They'll count the instruments and lap pads a couple of times during surgery to make sure that nothing is left inside your body. A retained foreign object (RFO) is listed as one of the "Never 27" events: the goal is that they should never happen. In an emergency situation where the scrub tech and nurse do not have time to count everything before the surgery starts, you will need an x-ray to confirm that there are no instruments, lap pads, or needles left behind inside your body before they finish closing everything up.

SYMPTOM	WHAT IT MEANS
Can't breathe	If you can talk, you can breathe. Try to figure out if the sensation is from not feeling yourself breathe, or if you are breathing but feel like you are not getting enough oxygen. Check the pulse oximeter to monitor your oxygen saturation.
Tingling fingers	You're as numb as you can get—the highest your anesthesia will go.
Numb lips	Sign of high blood level of local anesthetic or hyperventilation.
Feeling nauseous	Check blood pressure first. Could be impending low BP if right after the anesthesia. After baby is delivered, nausea is likely due to peritoneal tugging.
Going to pass out	Right after spinal/epidural block, impending hypotension (low BP). Check BP.
Shaking	Cold sensation, hormones, heat redistribution. Very Common. RX warm blanket, hot air blower, warmed IV fluids.
Feel numb	The anesthesia is working.

Figure 7. 1

Nip/Cut

Sometimes during a C-section, the bladder may tear or be "nicked" or cut. One non-specific sign of bladder wear and tear is blood in the urine. Instead of being clear or yellow, your urine can turn pinkish or even bloody. While a little bit of blood is frequent, typically from direct manipulation of the bladder by the surgeon or even by the baby's head, more blood is a worrisome sign.

If your surgeon thinks there might be a tear in the bladder, you may hear them talk about a blue dye. By filling the bladder with blue dye, it is easy to see if there is a leak of blue fluid out of the bladder and into the surrounding areas. The agent is methylene blue or indigo carmine, and it is either given by IV or injected directly into your bladder via the Foley catheter.

Bladder tears can be easily repaired with some suturing. Bigger ruptures may require a specialist and a urine catheter until the bladder heals. By the way: blue dye and yellow urine makes green, so if you're peeing green, don't worry! It's all a part of the plan.

Watch the Clock

How long does it take to get the baby out? Many women ask me this question. Usually it's about 3-5 minutes from the skin incision—the moment surgery actually starts. You will probably hear this event called out in the OR ("Skin!" or "Incision!") so that the nurses can record it.

If you've had a prior cesarean or prior abdominal surgery, there may be scar tissue, which will make the process a little longer. Women who have more tissue to go through because of a condition like obesity will also find that it takes longer for the OB to get the baby out.

The baby is typically not monitored during the surgery. The normal external ultrasound probe that is strapped to your belly cannot be used during surgery, as it would be in the surgical field. In some circumstances, the baby may already have an "internal" electrode—a FSE or fetal scalp electrode—usually due to difficulties with the fetal heart tracing. Some OBs remove the electrode before the surgery, while others continue to monitor the baby via the FSE during surgery. If there have been dips in the fetal heart rate, it's not a bad idea to keep it on until delivery. The baby's heart rate is the best way to monitor how he or she is tolerating what's going on.

Orientation Time

One reason there may be a slight delay or difficulty is if the baby is in a certain position. The way the baby is oriented is important. If you pushed for two hours and the baby did not come out vaginally, the head of the baby is probably wedged into your cervix and vaginal canal. Someone may actually have to push the baby's head up via the vaginal canal so the OB can pull the baby out! If the baby is lying in a transverse position, meaning across your belly left to right instead of head down in the cervical area, that can also make things difficult. The baby's body and head will need to be rotated around so the head is oriented directly down toward your pelvis.

You may hear other terms being used that refer to the fetal position. We already described the baby's head being wedged into the pelvis; the opposite is called "floating," where the head is able to move around. This position is not uncommon during a scheduled cesarean, and OBs generally like it because it's easy to pull the baby out. Then of course there's breech, which will almost always necessitate a cesarean as few OBs are willing to take the risk of a vaginal breech delivery.

A Double Setup

If you're expecting twins or triplets, welcome to the commotion—double your pleasure, double your fun! If you're having multiples, you'll almost always have a cesarean. If the babies are in a favorable position (e.g. vertex/vertex), some OBs may attempt a vaginal delivery, but always in the OR. That way, you'll deliver the first baby vaginally and, depending on how it goes, everyone is prepared to do a crash cesarean on the second baby if needed. It's a double setup. With multiples babies, expect lots of staff to help take care of them, causing a lot of noise and commotion – entirely normal.

The term "double setup" refers to being ready for both vaginal and cesarean deliveries. It's good to be prepared, because the placenta(s) can start to separate after the birth of the first baby. If this happens, the second baby's heart rate will dip, and a crash cesarean might be necessary. Most OBs will advise you to have an epidural in place—that way you can be awake and it's safer for you and your babies.

Early Arrivals

Premature babies are almost always delivered by cesarean, and this is a good thing—very premature babies (<25 weeks) have been reported to do better being born by cesarean.[i] During a cesarean there is less trauma to the head, and babies born prematurely have heads that are bigger in proportion to their bodies and therefore more susceptible to injury. However, the uterus is also smaller and may necessitate a classical incision on the uterus to make enough room to take the baby out. Sometimes the OB will request that the anesthesiologist give some Nitroglycerin to help relax the

> **INSIDER SECRET**
>
> Your red blood cells contain hemoglobin, which is what binds to the oxygen in your lungs, releasing the oxygen to your body's tissues. A young, healthy pregnant woman with a normal hemoglobin (e.g. 12 g/dL) can lose half of her blood volume—about 3 liters—and still have enough hemoglobin to carry oxygen around. Many practitioners refer to hematocrit ("crit"), which refers to the percent of the blood volume occupied by red blood cells. The simple conversion is 3:1. That is hematocrit 36 to hemoglobin 12.

uterus and ease the amount of pushing/pulling during delivery. Premature newborns are very fragile!

If you are at 28 weeks or less, oxytocin may be ineffective in causing the uterus to contract and stop bleeding because your body will not have produced many oxytocin receptors yet. You may need one of the direct-acting medications to help the uterus contract—either Methergine or Hemabate.

True Blood

Blood loss ends up mattering a good deal when you have a cesarean, so let's talk about it for a moment—what it means, what to look for, and how to prepare yourself so that bleeding doesn't cause you unnecessary stress or panic. This is blood, the *true* story.

When people think about blood, they generally think about the red stuff. But there are different components to blood, as well as different ways to keep up your blood volume in order to maintain your blood pressure and the perfusion of oxygen to your body.

Crystalloid and Colloid Solutions

Crystalloid (salt water) and colloid (starch or protein water) can be given to you to make up for blood loss. While these types of fluid do not themselves carry oxygen, they do provide volume for your heart to pump blood around. Common crystalloid solutions include saline (also called normal saline, or 0.9 NS), lactated ringers (also called LR), and Plasmalyte. Common colloid solutions include the starches, manufactured Hetastarch (Hespan and Hextend) and albumin (separated from human blood; either 5 percent or 25 percent solution). You need three times as much volume of crystalloid as colloid to replace an equal amount of blood volume lost. So in a bleeding pinch, colloid is a better replacement.

Normal vs. Abnormal

The normal amount of bleeding during a C-section can be almost a liter! At least, that's the number often quoted. Some of that is amniotic fluid—what the baby is floating in. I find that the typical blood loss is usually more like 700 ml. Not to worry—you can easily handle that amount of blood loss. Remember that one of the first normal physiologic changes in pregnancy is an increase in your blood volume, partly to prepare and compensate for bleeding after delivery. See? Your body is already taking care of you, and it's doing a nice job. For thousands of years women gave birth without doctors and without cesareans; they had to survive without blood transfusions or even medicine to help stop the bleeding.

But today's remarkable medical advancements don't hurt, especially when something goes wrong in the OR. Some women bleed a little more than they should when it's time for the baby to come. Very commonly this is due to placenta previa, which I mentioned earlier—the placenta is covering the opening from the cervix into the uterus. When this happens, blood can often leak or gush from the placenta-uterus interface.

A placenta previa has increased risk of being abnormally implanted into the uterus, which is called placenta accreta. If the placenta has implanted into the uterus deeper than normal, the muscle of the uterus can't contract properly and stop the bleeding when the placenta is removed. Placenta accreta usually winds up requiring a hysterectomy to stop the bleeding. Being familiar with these terms will save you valuable time and mental energy if an emergency arises. You don't have to be afraid, because you've already been clued into what is going on and what might happen.

Estimated Blood Loss

To make sure that you aren't losing more blood than normal, your doctor will want to figure out your EBL, or estimated blood loss. This can be tricky to determine as blood loss is typically underestimated.[ii] According to the American College of Obstetricians and Gynecologists, EBL is "notoriously inaccurate, with significant underreporting."[iii]

To tip the scales in the other direction, you and your partner should be clued in as to what to look for. In order to estimate the blood loss, you have to consider several areas. The suction canister will fill with blood *and* amniotic fluid, so the amount of amniotic fluid has to be estimated and subtracted from the total in the suction canister. An elective cesarean with a normal amount of amniotic fluid can amount to 300 cc. Also, just before closing the abdomen, the surgeon may irrigate the abdomen with salt water (normal saline), so you have to read the suction canister *before*. The lap pads have to be counted as well—not just the number of lap pads used (typically ten to twenty), but also how soaked they are. A fully soaked lap pad can hold 125 ml of blood (though they're usually not fully soaked).

Other places to look for an accurate EBL include the surgical drape, which usually has a pocket on each side to catch fluid and other "stuff." And don't forget to look on the floor. Sometimes the drapes are not well-applied and fluid leaks onto the floor or beneath the drape and onto the OR table beneath the patient. You can also find blood clots between the legs and within the uterus. This is why at the end of surgery, they "express" the uterus by pushing on it to expel any blood or blood clots. Retained blood clots can prevent the uterus from fully contracting down.

Several years ago, we encountered a situation with EBL at one of the hospitals where I was supervising. "Maria," a forty-year-old woman, had labored all day. But despite her best efforts and those of her OB, the baby did not want to drop down, or descend. The OB suspected the baby might be a bit big, but Maria wanted to try for a vaginal delivery.

After eighteen hours of labor, Maria went to cesarean section. The surgery progressed well, and the OB was right—the baby was over 9 pounds! There seemed to be a bit more blood loss than usual, but the suction canister showed 900 ml, which is not atypical. However, this was not a scheduled cesarean, and Maria had been in labor with her membranes ruptured (bag of water broken), meaning there wasn't the typical amniotic fluid diluting the blood in the suction canister. There were also extra packs of lap pads that were soaked and hanging in the corner.

So the OB estimated that the blood loss was slightly above average . . . but he only estimated it at 1000 ml. It was clear to me that the true blood loss was higher. Maria's heart rate was fast, ranging from 110 to 140 beats per minute. While her fever accounted for some of that, her high pulse was an indicator of low blood volume.

Rather than argue with the OB over exact blood loss, I gave colloid fluid to Maria, which helped bring the heart rate down. Then I checked a STAT hematocrit and other labs as soon as we arrived in the PACU (post anesthesia care unit—more on that in Chapter 8). Sure enough, Maria's hematocrit (blood count) had dropped by nearly half and she needed a blood transfusion of PRBC (red blood cells, see below).

Moral of the story: even skilled people can underestimate the blood lost during surgery. Studies have proven that blood loss is often underestimated by *everyone*, which is dangerous for you. It may be better to use clinical markers like heart rate, blood pressure, perfusion of skin (pink or white, sweaty) instead of relying on visual estimation.[iv] Always check a hematocrit anytime you have even the slightest question about whether you've lost too much blood. The only way to know for sure is to check.

For more information go to www.SafeBabySystem.com.

Open for Donations

If you are losing blood, you may need to receive Packed Red Blood Cells (PRBC), colloquially referred to as "blood." Receiving one unit of

PRBC will typically raise your hematocrit by 3. If you need blood, you will usually need two or more units (one donor, about 300 ml of blood).

The preferred blood to give is blood that has been "cross-matched," against your blood, thus making sure you don't have a reaction to the blood you receive. The cross-match process takes about 45 minutes, with the blood bank already having a sample of your blood (sometimes they want two!) and the proper paperwork. If there is no time, you can always receive O negative blood—the universal donor—as it does not have the major antigen molecules that people can react against. Either way, they should give you irradiated blood, which kills the donor white blood cells, preventing them from attacking your body (graft versus host reaction).

If you have a known medical problem where you will likely need blood during your cesarean (e.g., placenta accreta), you may arrange for autologous transfusion—where you donate blood for yourself ahead of time. That way you're actually receiving your own blood! The need for this is very uncommon, but it can be done. Just make sure you have enough time to make new blood before your cesarean—typically four weeks with great nutrition and iron supplementation.

You can also encourage your friends and family to go to the hospital and donate blood in your name—as long as they have the same or compatible blood type. This is called donor-directed blood. Most blood banks need three to seven days to process the blood and have it ready for donor-directed use. If you have family and friends who are interested in donating, have them go in beforehand, as it's too late if they go in on the day you need it.

If you are worried about needing a transfusion, at risk for needing a blood transfusion, or just interested, read the following section, otherwise, skip to page 122, *Postpartum Hemorrhage: What You Can Do.*

Care to Clot?

When you bleed a significant amount—say half your blood volume or more—you need to have more of the plasma components of the blood that help you form blood clots. These are called "clotting factors." The recent trend has been to give clotting factors like FFP earlier than in the past as a way of making sure you do not get into a downward spiral of bleeding due to a lack of clotting components, which is known as "wash out." You might also suffer from DIC (disseminated intravascular coagulation), a process that physiologically starts from a different path but winds up in the same predicament: not enough clotting components to make a clot.

There are four components that you may need to help with blood clotting: FFP, cryo, platelets, and Factor VII.

1. FFP

FFP, fresh frozen plasma, has most of the enzymatic clotting components you need to form a blood clot. There are over a dozen individual factors that compose the clotting cascade, and FFP contains nearly all of them. How much you receive depends on how much blood you have lost and the conditions of the surgical field—whether things are under control or bleeding and oozing. If you receive FFP, it's usually at least two units. The most recent recommendation, based on the military trauma literature, suggests using FFP from the start at an almost 1:1 ration to PRBC.

2. Cryo

Cryoprecipitate is also made from donor blood, but it is highly concentrated in fibrinogen, a key blood clotting factor that can be depleted. Usually when you receive cryoprecipitate, it is pooled from several donors so you get enough to boost your fibrinogen level.

3. Platelets

Platelets play a key role in initiating clot formation. Typically you have a lot of platelets circulating around, and have enough for even a moderate blood loss. That's why platelets are less frequently given, unless you're losing massive amounts of blood or you have a specific problem like DIC. Some medicines like aspirin will affect platelet function (that's why they give it to prevent heart attacks), which in turn decreases the ability to form blood clots. Platelets are also commonly pooled so you get the equivalent to, say, five people's platelets from their blood donation. It's even better if they give you a pheresis pack: lots of platelets from a single donor.

4. Factor VII

A new treatment for major blood loss is recombinant Factor VII. This factor also plays a key role in blood clot formation and has been recommended by many as being helpful in extreme blood loss. Unfortunately, Factor VII costs thousands of dollars and may not be available in all hospitals.

How safe is blood transfusion? Many women ask me this question. Thankfully, the answer is, "Very safe." When I started out in medicine, we did not know the cause of GRIDS (before it was called AIDS, it was GRIDS), and we went very far out of our way to avoid transfusions, a known cause of transmission. However, they now perform not just one, but several tests on donated blood to screen out blood tainted with infectious viruses like HIV, CMV, Hepatitis C, and more.

Today, the overall risk of getting infected is less than one in 100,000.[vi] If you are bleeding, the risk of injury or death is much greater than the risk of infection, so take the blood!

Time for Transfusion

If you need a blood transfusion, there are several steps to follow to ensure that you stay safe. The blood comes with an attached slip, so two nurses or doctors must cross-check that the blood is assigned to you. Remember: there may be patients with similar names or medical numbers in the hospital, and you want to make sure you've got the right blood. While this step may seem mundane, it's crucial for your safety—transfusing the wrong blood is one of the leading causes of complications from blood transfusions. In the United Kingdom, a shocking 60 percent of transfusion-related adverse events were due to the incorrect blood being transfused.[vii]

> **INSIDER SECRET**
>
> Your old friend calcium is good for more than just strong bones. Calcium is a key component to proper blood clotting. Most blood banking uses a calcium binder (chelator) to prevent the stored blood from clotting. If you're having bleeding problems or are receiving rapid transfusions, make sure you are getting extra calcium by IV, too!

The nurse will also check the expiration date, blood type, blood product serial number, and your birth date. Preferably the blood should go through a filter, which filters out unnecessary components that do not benefit you and may cause minor harm.

When you're experiencing rapid blood loss, you can easily lose 100 mL/minute. The right tools can save the day—not to mention your life. Having a working large-bore IV and the proper equipment to help transfuse you with warmed fluid can make the difference between a bad situation well-handled and the kind of high-ratings drama you see on *Grey's Anatomy*. Equipment like a rapid transfuser that can pressurize the bags of crystalloid, colloid, or blood while warming them can literally be a lifesaver.

If you know you're at risk for a bleeding complication of pregnancy, you should probably have two large-bore IVs in place before the surgery starts (either an 18-gauge IV, or possibly the large 16-gauge). Although

INSIDER SECRET

If you are at risk for bleeding, start the cesarean with two large bore IVs. No time to start messing around looking for a vein when you actually start bleeding – you need everyone to be focused on giving blood volume replacements.

it's a minor inconvenience, it's better to be safe. Once you start to bleed, it can be difficult to find a vein, and if your blood volume is low, your veins will be collapsed. A central line—a catheter placed in your neck or groin—is much more invasive and difficult to place, although sometimes necessary for intravenous access.

If you skipped the prior sections on blood replacement, you'll want to continue reading here…

Postpartum Hemorrhage: What You Can Do

Why am I spending so much time explaining blood and blood products? The answer is simple: because 140,000 women die every year worldwide from pregnancy related bleeding.[viii] This is called PPH, or postpartum hemorrhage.

Not only is hemorrhage one of the Big Three—embolism, hemorrhage, and preeclampsia; it is the *leading* cause of maternal death worldwide. What's sad is that, of these three dangers, hemorrhage is the most treatable and potentially avoidable. Prompt recognition and aggressive fluid and blood replacement can literally mean the difference between life and death.

Between 1994 and 2002, postpartum hemorrhage increased by 30 percent in the United States, and maternal transfusions increased by 600 percent![ix] The PPH rate increased even more in 2001-2005 to 2.6 percent of all deliveries: over 105,000 women annually.[x] And 1.6 percent of women (that's 1/62!) receive blood to help during a postpartum hemorrhage.[xi]

If you've had extra bleeding in a prior pregnancy, your chances increase during your next delivery, whether vaginal or cesarean. PPH in a prior pregnancy increases your chances of having it again over three-fold. And of course, if you have a history of a bleeding disorder, that could also increase your chances for bleeding during or after delivery. But by far the most common cause for excessive bleeding is uterine atony, which accounts for 70 percent of postpartum hemorrhage.[xii]

Uterine atony occurs when the uterus won't shrink and clamp down. The main risk factor is prolonged labor and exposure to oxytocin, with more than twenty-four hours leading to increased risk. Other risk factors include anything that stretches the uterus too much (e.g., multiple babies, extra amniotic fluid), uterine infection (e.g., chorioamnionitis, fever, high fetal heart rate), physical abnormality of the uterus (e.g., Fibroids, bifid, "Y"-shaped uterus), medications (magnesium), or grand multiparity (e.g. fourth or fifth baby).

Of the factors that can lead to uterine atony, the two over which you have the most direct control are magnesium and oxytocin exposure. Magnesium is used intravenously for preventing seizures in preeclampsia and for stopping premature labor, but it also increases your chances of uterine atony. And how long you've been in labor affects how much you've been on oxytocin, which also affects your odds. If uterine atony does develop, make sure you promptly receive direct-acting medications to make your uterus contract—Methergine, Hemabate, or rectal Cytotec. Some newer, non-surgical approaches include balloon tamponade and emergency angiogram embolization, where they inject "glue" into the uterine arteries to the uterus to stop the bleeding.

> **INSIDER SECRET**
>
> Magnesium is a competitive calcium antagonist whose effect can be reversed by giving IV calcium. If you're not already getting calcium intravenously for blood loss, one gram can help treat uterine atony. Calcium serves to trigger contractions, and I've found it to be very helpful in circumstances when the other drugs are not working.

If none of these actions are successful, the OB will need to start tying off your uterine arteries on the path toward hysterectomy. No one wants an emergency hysterectomy, but it's sometimes the only way to save your life. Emergency hysterectomies are on the rise, perhaps because of long labors, the overuse of oxytocin and rise in repeat cesareans.

It could also have to do with an in increasingly older, more at-risk pregnant population. Many of today's moms have underlying medical problems that lead to higher rates of postpartum hemorrhage. And the correlation between PPH and hysterectomies is undeniable: one study found a 73 percent increase in hysterectomies due to postpartum hemorrhage.[xiii] Other factors include having had more than three children, especially by cesarean; as the number of repeat repeat C-sections climb, the chance for placenta accreta and hysterectomies increases, too. Mothers over thirty-five are also at greater risk.

The best way to avoid an emergency hysterectomy is to simply hope for the best and plan for the worst. Educating yourself about the danger signs associated with PPH can help keep you calm and safe. Figure 7.2 shows a table of possible treatment steps, progressing from simplest to most severe.

The good news is that you can triumph over bleeding in the delivery room, and for mom and baby to be just fine. When the staff and the equipment are up to snuff and the transfusion goes smoothly, all is well. I've watched it happen a thousand times.

Recently, on a rainy night, I was called to the hospital to help out during a "surge," or busy period (Labor & Delivery has its own ebbs and flows; some say the lunar cycles and changes in weather affect how many women go into labor). It was a busy night, and my antennae were up, just in case something were to go wrong. After overhearing a conversation by two of the OB residents, I checked on "Lori," a patient who had already had a cesarean section. Lori had "dumped" 800 ml of blood clots into the bed. Not good.

Treatment of Postpartum Hemorrhage

TREATMENT	DOSAGE	POSSIBLE SIDE EFFECTS
Oxytocin (Pitocin)	Minimum 20 units in the body – IV, IM	Transient drop in blood pressure
Methergine (methylergonovine)	0.2 mg IM, not IV	Nausea/vomiting, hypertension
Hemabate (carboprost, a prostaglandin F2alpha)	250 micrograms IM/IU (intrauterine)	Hypertension, asthma, shivering
Misoprostol (Cytotec) rectal OR Dinoprostone (a prostaglandin E2)	1000 micrograms	Nausea/vomiting, fever, shivering
Surgical "glue" that helps stop a bleeding area, e.g. Floseal	Apply to surgical wound	
Surgical tie-off of uterine artery, hypogastric artery		
Possible angiogram and embolization of the arteries, if available.		Transfer to Radiology, should be reasonably stable
Alternative: balloon tamponade (e.g. Bakri balloon) within the uterus		

Figure 7. 2

When I went to see Lori, she was looking pale and kind of sweaty—sure signs of being hypovolemic (low blood volume). So I ordered two units of PRBC and two units of FFP while we drew blood for a stat hematocrit (blood count) and coagulation studies. I brought the rapid transfuser into her room and quickly set it up. By the time the blood arrived, we were ready to go.

With the rapid transfuser, it took 6 minutes per unit to infuse through her 18-gauge IV. Within a half hour she was rock solid, and the rectal Cytotec—medicine she had received to help firm up the uterus and ward off uterine atony—had kicked in and the bleeding slowed down. After another few hours of close watching, the danger period was over, and Lori was able to go bond with her baby. Both mom and baby went home, happy and healthy together.

Without proactive, aggressive treatment and the proper equipment in place, things could have gone very differently for Lori. A mere fifteen-minute delay for equipment or blood and the blood loss could have led to problems clotting, leading to further blood loss. And without fast replacement via a rapid transfuser, severe hypotension with a potential for kidney damage and cardiac arrest could have occurred. Lori's happy ending was made possible by good preparation and a hospital that was ready to meet her needs. Make sure you pick a hospital for your cesarean where strategic key equipment is pre-positioned on the Labor & Delivery floor.

Avoiding an Embolism

In Chapter 4, we discussed embolisms as they pertained to prevention—how to ensure that you didn't encounter one in the months leading up to your delivery. Now we're talking about special events that might occur during and immediately after your cesarean. I want to instruct you on what to do in the heat of the moment if all signs point to an embolism.

Though postpartum hemorrhage is the number one cause of maternal death worldwide, embolism is the number one cause of maternal mortality in the United States.[xiv] Fortunately, the overall rate is relatively rare—only 2.3 deaths from embolism in every 100,000 deliveries. In its less severe form, embolism can cause sudden shortness of breath, bleeding problems, and cardiac arrest.

To review: the three types of embolism are air embolism, amniotic fluid embolism, and pulmonary (or thrombotic) embolism. We mostly want to talk about that last one, but let's take a moment to recap the other two and what they mean for you.

Air Embolism

During a C-section, the open uterus may entrain air into the veins. A large bolus of air (generally an estimated 60 ml), may cause an "air lock" and block blood flowing through the heart. If this happens, quick and simple CPR may break up the air bubble and allow you to recover.

> **INSIDER SECRET**
>
> Keep the head of the bed up slightly so the venous pressure at the uterus is positive. This helps prevent air entrainment and can help you avoid an air embolism.

Amniotic Fluid Embolism (AFE)

An amniotic fluid embolism occurs when the amniotic fluid that the baby is floating in enters your bloodstream and causes difficulty in breathing, a drop in blood pressure, and cardiovascular collapse. The one sign that can mean nothing else but AFE is sudden onset of bleeding everywhere, or DIC. Treatment at this point is "supportive," aimed at restoring blood pressure, oxygen, ventilation, and replacing blood and clotting factors.

According to the classical literature, there's a 50 percent chance of death once AFE occurs. But with aggressive, rapid treatment, you can survive it. Take the story of "Mischa," a woman who was having a speedy labor during vaginal delivery when the fetal heart rate took a turn for the worse. Suddenly, Mischa had a seizure. We all rushed into her room to help and, with supportive measures, the seizure stopped. But the baby's heart rate dropped and we had to rush back for a crash cesarean. Because her blood pressure was high and we had no time, Mischa received general anesthesia. When the baby came out needing some resuscitation, I went to help.

A couple of minutes later, I checked with my resident to see how Mischa was doing. He sheepishly told me there was no carbon dioxide tracing, meaning that she was not perfusing her lungs. I immediately went to Mischa and gave her epinephrine to boost her heart and blood pressure. After aggressive therapy with medication and fluids, her blood pressure returned to normal, but she was bleeding everywhere—a sure sign of amniotic fluid embolism. But after receiving blood and FFP, her condition stabilized, and we were able to take her to the ICU. Mischa left the hospital awake, alert, and healthy, in spite of her near-death episode with AFE.

Pulmonary Embolism (PE)

Pulmonary embolism is the term used most commonly to mean thrombotic pulmonary embolism: a blood clot from the veins in the legs or pelvis that travels to the heart and lungs. When this happens, you can experience shortness of breath, high pulse rate, a drop in blood pressure, or sudden cardio-pulmonary arrest. Of the three types of embolism, this is the one that is the most preventable. In fact, a new trend in obstetrics is to take a more aggressive stance about trying to prevent pulmonary embolisms.

So what can you do to help prevent a PE from occurring post-op? The main reasons blood clots occur in your legs is due to low flow. Since the main source of blood clots is from the legs, you can increase the flow of blood by keeping your leg muscles moving. The leg muscles help pump the blood up, against gravity, out of the legs and into your body again. A classic reason people get a PE is because they were on a long plane or car ride and their legs were bent and not moving.

> **INSIDER SECRET**
>
> Even if you are in bed lying down, you can pump your calf muscles and feet against the footboard at the end of the bed. This will keep your muscles in shape and the blood moving around preventing blood clots in the legs.

But obviously, you can't exactly hop up and run around the room when you're numb and groggy after a C-section—and certainly not during one! One way to "trick" your body into thinking that you're moving is to wear progressive compression stockings, often called TED hose, to keep the veins small and help blood flow move out of the legs. Before your surgery, the nurses should place boots on your legs called SCDs (sequential compression device) that intermittently pump up and squeeze your calves and thighs to help move the blood pumping around, just as if you were using your legs. Ideally, you'll keep the SCDs on throughout surgery, continuing into the immediate post-op period.

In the event that you can't prevent a PE, you can certainly recognize the signs of one. If you feel sudden shortness of breath, fast heart rate, dizziness, or weakness, or if your partner feels the color in your face has changed (ashen is a sign of poor perfusion), call your nurse or doctor immediately. Early treatment can save your life.

Heparin is sometimes given prophylactically to prevent blood clots from forming, typically in the form of an injection into the skin once or twice daily. If you've been given LMWH (low molecular weight heparin) before your C-section, be sure to tell your anesthesiologist. You need to be off LMWH for twenty-four hours before getting an epidural or spinal. In fact it's best to switch from LMWH to regular heparin (twice a day dose) a couple of weeks before your expected delivery time. Regular heparin does not interfere with getting a regional anesthetic at the typical prophylactic dose. Also, just be aware that if you receive four days of heparin during postpartum recovery, you can infrequently develop a low platelet count due to HIT (heparin induced thrombocytopenia).

Though the studies are still in their earliest stages, heparin is proving to be an excellent way of combating pulmonary embolism. Since they've begun to put these post-operative measures in place, early reports from the UK show a 40 percent reduction in maternal deaths to PE. It's a two-step process: prevention first, and then, if that proves unsuccessful, early recognition can save the day.

* * *

So you made it! Emergency averted, disaster deterred. You've survived your C-section and are on the road to recovery. Now let's talk about what happens from the moment the doctor finishes sewing you up—beginning with the joy of holding your newborn baby in your arms.

Things To Keep In Mind

- Most C-sections go smoothly; in the event of problems, the more knowledgeable you are, the more prepared you'll be and the less fear you'll experience.

- If the surgeon talks about blue fluid (methylene blue or indigo carmine), he is probably concerned about a bladder tear, which can easily be repaired with some suturing.

- One reason there may be a slight delay or difficulty in getting the baby out is if the baby is in certain positions (e.g. transverse, wedge into the pelvis).

- If you're having multiples, you'll almost always have a cesarean.

- The normal amount of bleeding during a C-section can be almost a liter!

- Blood loss is typically underestimated.

- You can also encourage your friends and family to go to the hospital and donate blood in your name a week before—as long as they have the same or compatible blood type.

- Blood transfusion is very safe today.

- If you know you're at risk for a bleeding complication of pregnancy, you should probably have two large-bore IVs in place before the surgery starts.

- Postpartum hemorrhage is the leading cause of maternal death worldwide, but it is also the most preventable cause. Older mothers or women with underlying medical problems are more prone to postpartum hemorrhage.

- Aggressive treatment can prevent embolisms, or blood clots, from causing death.

- Heparin is proving to be an excellent way of combating pulmonary embolism.

Go to **www.SafeBabySystem.com/bonus** for additional information.

REFERENCES

[i] Malloy MH. Pediatrics 2008:122:285-92. Impact of cesarean section on neonatal mortality rates among very preterm infants in the United States, 200-2003.

[ii] Oyelese Y, Ananth CV. Postpartum hemorrhage: epidemiology, risk factors, and causes. Clin Obstet GYnecol 2010:53:147-156.

[iii] ACOG Practice Bulletin Clinical Management Guidelines For Obstetrician—Gynecologists Number 76, October 2006 *(Replaces Committee Opinion Number 266, January 2002)* Postpartum Hemorrhage.

[iv] Leduc D. Active management of the third stage of labour: prevention and treatment of postpartum hemorrhage. J Obstet Gynaecol Can 2009:10:980-93.

[v] Fuller AJ, Bucklin BA. Blood product replacement for postpartum hemorrhage. Clin Obstet Gynecol 2010:53:196-208.

[vi] Ibid.

[vii] Fuller AJ, Bucklin BA. Blood product replacement for postpartum hemorrhage. Clin Obstet Gynecol 2010:53:196-208.

[viii] Oyelese Y, Ananth CV. Postpartum hemorrhage: epidemiology, risk factors, and causes. Clin Obstet Gynecol 2010:53:147-156.

[ix] Oyelese Y, Ananth CV. Postpartum hemorrhage: epidemiology, risk factors, and causes. Clin Obstet Gynecol 2010:53:147-156.

[x] Berg CJ. Obstet Gynecol 2009113:1075-81. Overview of maternal morbidity during hospitalization for labor and delivery in the United States 1993-1997 and 2001-2005.

[xi] Fuller AJ, Bucklin BA. Blood product replacement for postpartum hemorrhage. Clin Obstet Gynecol 2010:53:196-208.

[xii] Oyelese Y, Ananth CV. Postpartum hemorrhage: epidemiology, risk factors, and causes. Clin Obstet Gynecol 2010:53:147-156.

[xiii] Oyelese Y, Ananth CV. Postpartum hemorrhage: epidemiology, risk factors, and causes. Clin Obstet Gynecol 2010:53:147-156.

[xiv] CDC MMWR, Pregnancy-Related mortality surveillance –United States, 1991-1999, MMWR Surveillance summaries, February 21, 2003/52(SS02);1-8.

PART III
RECOVERING FROM A CESAREAN

Additional Bonus Materials are being created just for you.
As a special thank you, go to
www.SafeBabySystem.com/bonus

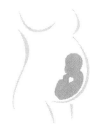

Chapter 8

In the PACU: Road to Recovery

Congratulations! After your OB puts in the final staples or sutures, your surgery is officially over. Your C-section is a thing of the past; now all that's left is recovery . . . and, of course, basking in the joy of your new little bundle.

So what do you do next? How can you function when it hurts? And what can you do to speed up recovery?

You've come to the right place. In the following chapters, we'll talk about what happens after that final stitch. Pay careful attention, because you won't find a lot of these tips anywhere else—learn how to have a faster, easier, less painful recovery so you can do what matters most—enjoy your baby.

Cleaning Up and Moving Out

Depending on the hospital's policies, you may be able to hold your baby in the OR during the surgery. You'll need someone to place your baby on your chest and help to support him or her. I'll often remind the dad or partner to use one hand to help stabilize the baby on mom's chest while taking pictures with the other hand.

Some women feel too weird or uncomfortable being flat to hold the baby. No worries. You can hold your baby when you sit up after the surgery. You won't miss out on any pivotal mother-baby bonding time.

Sometimes the nurses may want to take the baby to the nursery before the surgery is over. You and your labor partner have to decide where he or she is going to go: to stay with baby or with mom. If everything has been going well so far, it's okay for your partner to go with the baby to the nursery. If there is any doubt about what's been going on during surgery—for example, if there's been excessive bleeding or any unusual signs or symptoms—then it may be better to stay with mom until she goes to the recovery room and things seem stable. Remember: your labor partner is your extra pair of eyes and ears, looking out for your well-being when you may be too tired or groggy to do so.

After the OB is finished and the surgery is over, the circulating nurse and scrub tech will clean you up. You should just hug your arms across your chest and they will turn you side to side so they can clean both sides of your back. When they're finished, they'll put a clean sheet (or chux disposable pad) under you.

INSIDER SECRET

When using a roller board, make the OR table a smidge taller and tilt it to make for an easier, smoother transfer. It's easy on the back, too.

Now hold on for a ride! As your anesthesia probably hasn't worn off yet and won't for another hour or two, the surgical team will move you from the OR table to the stretcher. Either three to four people will help move you over, or they will use a roller board to move you.

After you get onto the stretcher, it's going to feel a lot better for you if your head is raised. All that extra blood that was going to your head will drain and you will feel less congested. You may even be allowed to hold your baby on the way to the recovery room.

A word to your labor partner: it's your job to be on "monitoring alert" during transfer from the OR. If mom is sleepy, make sure that she has oxygen in transport. Better yet, keep talking to her; make sure she is awake and responsive. Trouble can happen at this stage if sedation was given to mom. If she's awake and talking, everything is fine. If she is too sleepy, you could be started down the short path to trouble.

Years ago, at a hospital in the south, a woman named "Harriet" had just given birth by C-section. The surgery was over and things seemed fine; the baby was healthy, and Harriet was tired but otherwise okay. She'd been in some pain during surgery and was given some extra medication—fentanyl and midazolam—to lessen her pain and help her to relax. So the nurses and surgical team moved her over to the stretcher. Then everyone turned around to collect their paperwork and clean up.

Suddenly, her husband exclaimed, "Are you there, honey?"

Everyone turned around to see Harriet, blue and not breathing!

The anesthesiologist immediately grabbed a mask and started to breathe for her. Fortunately, there was no significant time delay, and they were able to fully resuscitate her. A little extra vigilance can go a long way to keeping mom and baby safe, healthy, and alive!

In the Recovery Room

After your trip down the hall, you'll finally be in the recovery room, also known as the PACU (post anesthesia care unit). Welcome to your new home for the next little while. You should be hooked up to the monitors right away—ECG, blood pressure, and pulse oximetry. Many hospitals allow the baby to come with you to PACU so you can bond and breastfeed. Of course, both mom and baby need to be doing well for this to happen. Otherwise, baby will go to the nursery, and mom will get to be with her newborn when she gets to her postpartum room.

Your stay in the recovery room will depend on the following factors: how long it takes for the anesthesia to wear off, when another room is ready for you, and how stable you have been during surgery. Stability has to do with how much you are bleeding and how awake you are.

Common issues in the PACU include being nauseous, sleepy, shivering, checking for bleeding, recovering from the anesthesia, holding you baby, and family visits. Hospitals have differing policies about visitors in the PACU. It's helpful to remind your friends and families that, if they are allowed in, to remember the other patients, even in their moment of excitement. Also, having a cesarean, especially if following being in labor, is totally exhausting. You need some rest, too! Sleepiness is okay, but you should be looking and talking normally, and it shouldn't be hard for your labor partner or the nurses to rouse you. If not, alert your nurse. The nurse will also check that your uterus stays firm and that you are not bleeding, either vaginally or into your abdomen. A little Lochia (bleeding vaginally) is normal, like a very heavy menstruation. Your uterus may even be massaged in order to help it stay firm. Your urine output will be checked hourly.

> **INSIDER SECRET**
>
> Remember to keep the lights on in the PACU. You need to be constantly assessed to make sure you look pink and perfused, not pale and sweaty (signs of low perfusion or blood pressure).

Shivering after a cesarean is very common. It's also a nuisance. Some shivering may be unavoidable; even women who deliver vaginally without any anesthesia shiver after giving birth! We're still not sure exactly why—possibly due to hormonal factors. However, shivering after a C-section has additional contributing factors. The OR is usually cold, which can lower your temperature. Sometimes the anesthesia can affect your body's temperature regulation and thermal set point, so your measured temperature drops and you shiver. And as if you needed any more potential reasons: some medications, like the prostaglandins used to help the uterus contract (e.g., Hemabate), are known to cause shivering and nausea.

Staying warm is particularly important in the PACU, and not just for comfort—for your health. You want to be especially wary of infection during the recovery period. If the recovery room is warm, it supports the functioning of your white cells that fight infections. Practically all the processes going on in your body are controlled by enzymes, and enzyme function is dependent upon temperature. As your temperature drops, the enzyme reactions slow down. These reactions slow down an estimated 10 percent for every 1°C decrease.[i] Keeping yourself warm will ensure that your body is functioning and repairing at top speed.

What can you do about it? If you're following the instructions in this book, you already asked the doctors to keep the OR warm during your surgery. Ask the same for the PACU. Cover up with a warm blanket to conserve heat. You can even get a forced air blanket to blow hot air on you, or a fancy new electric blanket can be placed under you. An isolated side effect of a classic pain medicine—Demerol, also called meperidine—can also help stop shivering. But since it's a narcotic, Demerol will contribute to making you a bit sleepy, too.

If you are shivering, the automated blood pressure cuff will have a difficult time taking your blood pressure. As the machine gets confused by arm movement, it pumps up tighter, and can hurt. I suggest trying to hold your arm still and straight when the machine is taking your blood pressure. If you can't hold your arm still, try putting the cuff on your leg. It still works; the number is just slightly higher.

If you are feeling faint, you want to check your blood pressure. After that, you may need to check your blood sugar. Many women have been in labor for hours, not eating or drinking, their bodies working just as hard as a marathon runner—if not harder. Add on top of that the stress of surgery, and the possibility of low blood sugar should come as no surprise.

A simple blood test, either by drawing blood or a finger prick, will quickly give you the answer. You can get sugar in the intravenous fluid, or even as a bolus of D50 (dextrose 50 percent), if your sugar is very low. Normal blood sugar is 80 mg/dL or above.

You'll want to keep an eye out for infections in the recovery room. Preventing infections is an easy way to help avoid a prolonged stay in the hospital. You should be alert to omissions of sterile technique; feel free to point them out. These include people coming into the room wearing long sleeves that are under the scrubs, touching something unsterile during a procedure and not changing gloves, and injecting through the IV without wiping with alcohol. Also, workers who appear obviously sick—e.g., sneezing and runny nose—should not be working if they're contagious.

Hand-washing is the latest hot topic—not everyone washes their hands enough. The current recommendation is for everyone to wash their hands or use alcohol-gel before and after *every time they touch you*. If a nurse or aide is about to touch you and you noticed they haven't washed their hands, you can offer a polite reminder by asking, "Would you like some Purell?"

No PPH in the PACU

Speaking of blood . . . let's take a moment to revisit postpartum hemorrhage. You're not out of the woods yet. Bleeding can occur anytime from right after the birth to several hours later. That's why it is imperative that you (and your labor partner) are alert for bleeding for the first twenty-four hours after you deliver.

You might notice increasing pain in your belly, and that your abdomen seems to have increased in size—both of which might indicate internal bleeding. A high heart rate, especially above 120 beats per minute, indicates something more should be looked into, and that a hematocrit test needs to be taken immediately. Being pale in the face, fingernails, or edge of the eyelids also indicates poor perfusion or low blood count. If you feel faint like you might pass out, that, too, is another indicator of low blood volume.

A simple test you can do even without a nurse is called orthostatic hypotension. Check your pulse (and blood pressure, if you can) lying down, and again after 30 seconds of sitting up with your legs dangling, or even standing up. If your pulse increases more than 20 beats per minute, you might have a low blood volume.

Another way to see how you are doing is to monitor your urine output. You should be producing at least 30 mL/hr, and preferably more. If you aren't, it might be a sign that your blood volume, and thus delivery of blood to the kidneys, is low. When in doubt, check your hematocrit. And look for signs of bleeding somewhere. Keep in mind that it might not be obvious. If there are some signs of bleeding, make sure they also check the "coags"—ability of the blood to clot—while drawing blood for the complete blood count.

See Figure 8.1 to get an idea of the numbers you want to be looking for. Ask for the results and if the values are out of range, be sure to discuss with your nurse and doctor.

Common Blood Test Table of Bleeding/Coagulation Status in the PACU:

Hemoglobin	Normal 11-14 mg/dl pregnancy
Hematocrit	Normal 32-38 pregnancy
Platelets	Normal >150,000 in pregnancy
CBC	Complete blood count includes above
PT/PTT	PT 12-14 (INR 1.3)/ PTT 32-35 normal
Fibrinogen	300-500 mg/dL normal pregnancy
Urine output	>30 cc/hr minimum
Blood pressure (BP) *Systolic BP* *Diastolic BP*	>90 for most women; >140 means preeclampsia possible low not that important; >90 means preeclampsia possible
Pulse	Want >50 and <120 beats per minute. >120 requires evaluation for bleeding, infection, fever etc.

Figure 8.1

Tissue Integrity

Having personally helped over 24,000 women give birth, you might call me an expert in a somewhat unusual area. We all come in different shapes, sizes, and personalities, but there's one area in particular where I've noticed significant differences over the years, and that's tissue integrity.

The basic quality of your body—how it feels and looks; how resilient the tissue is to pinching, pushing, and to needle inserts and medication injections—is called tissue integrity. For such an important factor, it's poorly quantified and not very well studied at all. Some women simply have better tissue integrity and heal more rapidly than others.

I've seen women bleed more, have longer surgeries, and have a tougher time recovering, all because they have poor tissue integrity. One story in particular comes to mind. "Hannah" was a thirty-eight-year-old woman who labored for several hours and went to cesarean section for failure to progress. The baby came out fine, but the surgeon had difficulty when it came time to sew her up. I watched, with interest and then with fear, as stitch after stitch tore through Hannah's tender tissues. The medical term for this is "friable"—when the tissue just tears and crumbles.

The OB tried different sutures and needles of various sizes, and every time, it just kept tearing the tissues. In the meantime, Hannah kept "oozing" blood. After what seemed like an eternity, the surgeon was able to stop the blood loss and get the tissues close enough together so they could heal. However, just like on the surface of skin, if you have constant pulling and tugging on a former scar, the scar gets bigger and weaker. You can only imagine what happened to this poor woman's insides!

Since there's a lack of scientific evidence on what causes strong tissue integrity, the best you can do for now is to eat well, take your vitamins, drink plenty of clean water, and exercise. Don't forget to de-stress and sleep enough—your body releases growth hormone at the later stages of your sleep cycle, which is crucial for bodily repair. Also, make sure you're getting enough Vitamin C, a key component of the connective tissue matrix.[ii] More on vitamins in Chapters 9 and 10.

Discharge Criteria

Once things are going well and the nurses feel you're recovering the way they like to see, you'll get to leave the PACU and finally go to your postpartum room. The criteria for discharge include recovering from your spinal or epidural anesthesia—being able to move your legs, as well as being alert and having normal vital signs—blood pressure, pulse, breathing rate, and urine output.

When is it a bad idea to go to your postpartum room? When you need more attention, or a higher level of nursing care. Most postpartum floors are staffed at one nurse to eight patients. If you need close watching for possible bleeding, excessive sleepiness, or any other problem, you might need to go to either a "step-down" unit or the ICU. The bonus: you'll get more nursing attention and close watching as the ratios are a lot better. A step-down unit is typically one nurse to two patients, and an ICU unit is one nurse per patient.

If things have not gone as well as you would have liked during your cesarean, one splurge you might want to consider is hiring your own nurse for the first night. By hiring your own nurse, typically assisted through the nursing office of the hospital, you can have constant attention, pampering, and closer watching. Private duty nursing can be a registered nurse, or even a lower level helper who is not a nurse. What level of help you could benefit from depends on whether you are feeling weak and shaky, or if you just feel like having a little extra help.

* * *

So you've left the PACU and are headed to a private room. What can you look forward to, and what do you want to look out for? In the next chapter, we'll discuss the ins and outs of the postpartum room, and how to ensure that you'll be heading home with your baby the moment you're both safe and sound.

Things To Keep In Mind

- Depending on the hospital's policies, you may be able to hold your baby right in the OR during the surgery.

- Your stay in the recovery room (also called PACU – post anesthesia care unit) will depend on the following factors: how long it takes for the anesthesia to wear off, when another room is ready for you, and how stable you have been.

- Shivering after a cesarean is very common. It's also a nuisance. Tips to avoid shivering: keep the OR and PACU warm, use warmed fluids and hot air blower, a narcotic called meperidine can help stop shivering, albeit make you a little sleepy.

- If you are feeling faint, you want to check your blood pressure, pulse and blood sugar.

- If a nurse or aide is about to touch you and you noticed they haven't washed their hands, you can offer a polite reminder by asking, "Would you like some Purell?"

- Tissue integrity varies from person to person. Taking your vitamins can help.

- Once things are going well and the nurses feel you're recovering the way they like to see, you'll get to leave the PACU and finally go to your postpartum room.

- If things have not gone as well as you would have liked during your labor and/or cesarean, one splurge you might want to consider is hiring your own private duty nurse for the first night.

Go to www.SafeBabySystem.com/bonus for additional information.

REFERENCES

[i] Forbes S. et al. Evidence-Based Guidelines for Prevention of Perioperative Hypothermia. J Am Coll Surg 2009:209:492-503.

[ii] Ivanov V et al. Anti-atherogenic effects of a mixture of ascorbic acid, lysine, proline, arginine, cysteine, and green tea phenolics in human aortic smooth muscle cells. J Cardiovasc Pharmacol 2007:49:140-145.

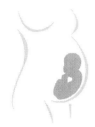

Chapter 9

In the Postpartum Room: The Final Stretch

The postpartum room is a quiet, safe haven, a place for you to heal and recover over the next few days. I've said it a dozen times, but I'll say it again: the more you know, the calmer, the more smoothly and faster your recovery will be. And the faster your recovery, the sooner you can focus on your baby! Just like at every other stage of the process, preparedness is key.

In this chapter, we'll talk about how to ensure your stay in the postpartum room is safe and comfortable so that you're back home in no time.

Can I Get You a Drink?

If your surgery went well, you can start to have clear liquids as soon as four hours after you've left the PACU. If you are thirsty before four hours, you can usually get a few ice chips to melt in your mouth and keep your lips and throat moist.

You're probably going to be thirsty—you may even have parched lips and a dry throat—and you'll want to drink to your heart's content. A word to the wise: once you can have fluids, go slow! Start with only a few sips at a time. If you drink too much too fast, it will likely make you nauseous.

You're not the only one who's thirsty; your baby wants a drink, too! Breastfeeding is encouraged by all the OB, pediatrics, and midwife organizations. Breastfed babies tend to be healthier and get fewer infections than bottle-fed babies. Make sure you're taking fish oil, or DHA, while breastfeeding. This will increase the DHA content in your breast milk, and DHA is critical for your baby's developing nervous tissue, including the brain and parts of the eyes. If you do decide to bottle feed your baby, make sure DHA is a component of the formula—studies have shown improved vision (visual acuity)[i] and fewer respiratory illnesses.[ii]

In addition to the benefits for your baby, your recovery will be faster, too. You generate a lot of calories by producing breast milk for the baby, which is good for your body. It's true: breastfeeding will actually help you lose pregnancy weight faster. Your uterine contractions will also be more intense than those in non-breastfeeding women because your body will be producing more oxytocin. In effect, your uterus will shrink more quickly as you recover. Now how's that for a deal?

If you are having trouble breastfeeding or not producing enough colostrum or milk, ask for a lactation consultation. Some mothers choose to supplement or exclusively use formula. For more information on the pros and cons of breastfeeding, see Chapter 13 of *The Safe Baby System.*

Move to the Groove

Doctors used to think that staying in bed for a week was good for you, but this theory no longer holds water. You may be sore and sleepy, but staying still in bed for days on end is actually bad for you! You want to be able to get up and have some movement in the first few hours after you get to your postpartum room—called early mobilization.

You don't need to do laps around the nurses' station. In fact, please don't! You'll want to take it easy. But many doctors and hospitals are having women get out of bed, even if only to go to the bathroom or a chair, on the first day after your cesarean. Even just taking a few steps is good for you. Some doctors or nurses will tell you to stay in bed for 24 hours after a spinal, but this is not necessary as studies have shown no difference in the chances of developing a 'spinal' headache.

Of course, if you've had more serious complications from the surgery, your doctor and nurse may tell you you're not allowed to get up and move around. For most women, though, a little move 'n groove is a good thing. By the second day after your cesarean, you want to be doing at least some slow walking around.

How can you move around if it hurts? Here's a trick that may be helpful: if you have to cough, sneeze, or move yourself from one side to the other—and especially when you get out of bed—use a pillow or your hands to press gently against your surgical wound. That way you won't have as much tension and movement at the site of the incision, and thus less pain. If you've been doing your core muscle exercises (abdominis transversus and pelvic floor) during your pregnancy, those muscles will become your best friends—a key aide in moving around and recovering faster. Dynamic, easy exercises will keep the core in shape —you shouldn't be doing abdominal crunches. It is also helpful to have good range of motion in your chest (thoracic spine) and hips. See video at www.SafeBabySystem.com/exercises.

As we discussed earlier, moving around will also help prevent you from getting a pulmonary embolism or deep vein thrombosis (which can often lead to a PE). Motion in your legs will also help move the muscles that pump the lymphatic system.

The lymphatic system is extremely important and regrettably under-appreciated. Even if you came into the hospital with your normal ankles, you can still get leg swelling. Actually, the swelling of your legs—indeed, of your whole body—will often get a little bit worse right after your cesarean. Think about it. You receive IV fluids for the anesthesia and surgery. But after the baby is born, all the blood that was going to the uterus and baby is now coming back to you. Your extremities are on overload!

Your body will start to "mobilize" the fluid in your tissues on its own, urinating it all out in one or two days, and may take a couple of weeks to return to normal. But why not help speed the process along? By increasing the movement in your legs and thus the movement of fluid through the lymphatic system, you'll help remove the excess fluid, decreasing the swelling. And who doesn't want their pre-pregnancy legs back? As an added side benefit, it helps to fight infection by moving the white blood cells around, too.

INSIDER SECRET

Creating your own exercise program for recovery can be fun. Keep it simple, low-key, and low-impact, and you'll be back on your feet in no time.

Even if you can't get up out of bed as much as you would like, you can still take steps that do almost as well. How? By pumping your legs . . . even if you're in bed!

It's true: just the action of pumping your legs can bring about the same positive effects as walking. You can gently push against the end of the bed with your feet. Do them together or one side and then the other—whatever works best for you. Do this for 5 minutes each leg, and repeat every two hours. Both a physical therapist and a personal trainer I consulted both suggest doing mini-squats to get into shape and maintain mobility of your hip and lower back. See video at www.SafeBabySystem.com/exercises.

And there's no harm in asking for a leg massage, either. It not only helps move the fluid into the lymphatic system and out of your legs . . . it feels good, too. A great job for your partner!

Take Your Vitamins

Your body is only as strong as the fuel you put into it. So why not boost it up with all the good stuff that will help you heal?

Here's a partial list of the vitamins and minerals you should be taking in the postpartum room: vitamin B5, vitamin C, copper, zinc, magnesium, and manganese, all of which help repair damaged tissue.[iii]

You also need a full complement of essential fats and essential amino acids. They work together. For example, you need extra vitamin C in addition to a couple of essential amino acids to produce connective tissue. Guess what you need the most to heal from surgery? That's right—connective tissue. One study showed stronger scar formation when given vitamin B5 and vitamin C for a week before minor skin surgery.[iv]

If you had staples placed, they'll generally take the staples out before you leave the hospital. Just be careful and don't pull or stretch across the incision for quite a while; doing so will increase the scar size. If you have the slow-dissolving sutures, nothing needs to be done—just avoid excess tension across the area. Having a good range of motion in your hips and chest help here, too. Certain vitamins have been shown to help scars heal faster; Coenzyme Q10 in particular has been suggested to help skin healing.[v]

And it isn't just you who benefits from taking vitamins. You need the full range of nutrients so that you not only heal, but are feeding your baby everything he or she needs by producing healthy breast milk.

Don't Be a Pain

Another important step toward early recovery is to take your pain medicine. The usual pain medications are safe for breastfeeding, but make sure to tell your nurse if you are breastfeeding or not. By taking your pain medicines, you will help yourself in the long term. By being relatively comfortable, you can move around, take deep breaths, and potentially help reduce long-term chronic pain. Remember that 10-18 percent of women who experienced significant pain after a cesarean suffered from chronic pain a whole year later.[vi]

There is definitely a correlation between the pain you experience in the postpartum room and any chronic pain that may develop later on. Women with pain at one year recalled more pain on postpartum day 1. In fact severe acute pain after surgery was associated with a more than double risk of having chronic persistent pain, and even postpartum depression.

INSIDER SECRET

If you're worried about becoming addicted to painkillers, don't be. Treating acute pain in the short term does not cause addiction. People only get "hooked" on pain medicines when they take them longer than the three to four days you are in the hospital, and typically with chronic problems like back pain.

Part of how chronic pain develops has to do with the spinal cord "wind up," meaning that once certain neural tracts in the spinal cord have been sensitized to the presence of pain, the pain gets "remembered," setting up a continuing cycle. Risk factors for chronic pain after cesarean include increased pain in the immediate post-op period or having pain present elsewhere (e.g., back pain, migraine), which can double your odds for chronic pain.[vii]

Don't be afraid to take your pain medication. Toughing it out is not the way to go anymore. By having good pain relief and employing preemptive analgesia, thereby preventing pain before it occurs, you can prevent spinal cord wind-up and drastically reduce your chances for chronic pain. It's better for you, both in the short term and the long term. Your body will thank you in the months to come.

You want to optimize the pain medicines you receive. Optimization begins by the right timing. If you are taking two pain medicines, do not take them together. You'll get much greater benefit if you stagger them. That way, they peak and wear off at different times, and you'll have more evenly distributed pain relief, avoiding too much when you first absorb them and too light right before your next dose. For example, if you were taking Vicodin and Motrin, you would want to take one and then the other two hours later.

By far the most common mainstay of pain relief after a C-section is epidural or spinal morphine. Given into your back, the morphine enters the spinal fluid and works for up to twenty-four hours, providing better quality pain relief than IV narcotics. If for some reason you didn't or couldn't get it, don't worry: you can get an IV PCA. PCA, or patient controlled analgesia, is when you can control all or part of the administration. The most common and safest way is when there is no basal infusion, and you control when you get the narcotic pain medicine, typically either morphine or Dilaudid (generic name: hydromorphone).

There are also newer, different methods of treating pain. Newer therapies include local anesthetic infusion into the surgical site, TAP blocks (transversus abdominal plexus), and continuous epidural infusion of dilute local anesthetic, usually with narcotic. The local anesthetic blocks the transmission of pain impulses to—you guessed it—your spinal cord. Remember: less pain and more movement means faster recovery. Not all hospitals offer these different medical therapies, though, and the ones that do don't always advertise them. So if you're interested, be sure to ask.

Alternative pain therapies are also a possibility, though they're not widely available in the USA. These include acupuncture, TENS, biofeedback, hypnosis, or EFT. Acupuncture has been used for thousands of years in Eastern medicine for treating diseases, as well as acute and chronic pain. TENS stands for transcutaneous electrical nerve stimulation, and is used to modulate neuroreceptors and block pain impulses in the spinal cord. Hypnosis has long been known to help reduce your perception of pain, improve anxiety, and even lessen nausea. EFT—emotional freedom technique—uses tapping along the meridians used in acupuncture, and has been reported to be helpful in pain states. For more on these and other alternative remedies, visit www.SafeBabySystem.com.

Speaking of pain: let's talk about headaches. Headaches aren't necessarily something to be worried about; you just have to make sure it's a common headache and not a harbinger of something more serious. If your headache is clearly positional—no or very little headache when you're lying flat, and quick onset of a severe headache when you sit or stand—then it's due to the spinal or epidural anesthesia causing post dural puncture headache (PDPH). It's convenient to get this taken care of while you are still in the hospital. If you have a severe positional headache, or if it's accompanied by blurry vision or buzzing in the ears, the PDHD will probably require an epidural blood patch. Speak to your anesthesiologist if you develop a positional headache.

Regular headaches are common postpartum. They can be from stress, not eating, caffeine withdrawal, or migraines. However, a constant severe headache needs to be brought to the attention of the hospital staff. You may need a CT scan of your head to makes sure you don't have a more dangerous condition—like a blood clot in the brain, cortical vein thrombosis, subdural hematoma, or subarachnoid hemorrhage. Fortunately, these bad events occur rarely—about 1/3000 or less. If you get the "worst headache of your life," you need to tell your nurse or doctor immediately.[viii]

Preventing Pneumonia

Outright pneumonia is not that common after cesarean, primarily because most women having babies are relatively young and healthy. You don't see a lot of seventy-five-year-olds with fragile lungs in Labor

& Delivery! However, you can take steps to help prevent pneumonia, which *is* one of the most common complications following surgery of any kind.

The medical term for preventing pneumonia is "pulmonary toilet." Not the nicest mental image, but it denotes a very good set of methods used to clear mucus and secretions from the airways. Pulmonary toilet means making sure you inhale deeply and cough up any gunk in your lungs. Many women come into L&D with a cold, especially during flu season. You are at increased risk for pulmonary complications like pneumonia if you are already sick when you come in, so this section is especially important for you.

After surgery, you want to take deep breaths, several times in a row, to expand your chest. During surgery you can have little areas of the lung that don't ventilate (exchange air) well; these can collapse in what is called atelectasis. If you don't clear the mucus in these areas, infection can develop. If you already have a cold, it's even worse, because these sites may already be infected by virus or bacteria.

Taking deep breaths and holding for a few seconds will help to reopen these areas of the lungs and can help you cough out the mucus that's down there. If you have a lot of congestion in your lungs, a breathing treatment may help you to bring up the gunk. I recommend an albuterol nebulizer (not the little hand-held pump). Breathing humidified air can moisten and help you to bring up the phlegm. Even saltwater (saline) mist or nasal spray can help you clear mucous and congestion from your nose and sinuses.

Special Precautions

Be familiar with your medical history—and any special challenges it presents—during your stay in the postpartum room. Certain diseases require extra caution and attention. Just so you're prepared, let's cover a couple of common diseases like diabetes, preeclampsia, and AMA.

Diabetes

If you have diabetes, whether gestational diabetes (brought on by pregnancy) or preexisting diabetes, the time for vigilance is not over. You still need to maintain tight control of your blood sugar after you deliver. If you are a long-term, insulin-dependent diabetic, you already know this. But even for gestational diabetes, you want to have tight control of your blood sugar in the period right after you deliver.

Remember those white blood cells that fight infection? Well, they get slowed down if your blood sugar is too high, which encourages infection. Many doctors specializing in diabetes want to continue tight management, which usually involves insulin infusion and close glucose monitoring for several hours after the birth. Beware of the signs of too low a blood sugar: feeling weak, shaky, sweaty, or just feeling generally bad.

INSIDER SECRET

Women who have developed preeclampsia during pregnancy have a higher chance of having high blood pressure and coronary artery disease later in life. And high blood pressure during pregnancy increases the risk of later developing hypertension by about 500 percent and diabetes by over 300 percent. If you've experienced either of these conditions, be sure to get close, long-term follow-up by your primary care internal medicine doctor or cardiologist. This could save your life.

Magnussen EB et al. Hypertensive disorders in pregnancy and subsequently measured cardiovascular risk factors. Obstet Gynecol 2009:114:961-70.

Preeclampsia

Although delivery of the baby and placenta is the true treatment for preeclampsia, the danger is not over after you deliver. You can first develop preeclampsia even 24 hours after you deliver. If you have preeclampsia, you will still be on magnesium post-delivery for seizure prevention, which can make you sleepy, nauseous, and weak. The blood level has to be carefully monitored. If you feel excessively sleepy or weak or are having difficulty breathing, alert your nurse right away! Your partner should be alert for these signs too. If your urine output decreases, you may need to have your magnesium turned off, as magnesium is eliminated via the urine.

Advanced Maternal Age (AMA)

No, "AMA" doesn't just stand for the American Medical Association. It can also mean Advanced Maternal Age, referring to an increase in the age at which women give birth to their first child. AMA is now a widespread phenomenon, especially in Western countries.

More and more women are waiting until later in life to have children. This can be a truly wonderful thing, as there are many benefits to waiting to have children. Older mothers can offer their children a sense of stability, emotional maturity, and financial security that many younger mothers cannot. Just keep in mind that your body is not as resilient at age forty as it was at age twenty. As we age, it takes longer to heal. That's why it becomes even more important to take care of yourself pre-pregnancy, during pregnancy, and after delivery.

It's especially important to be in good cardiovascular shape. Pregnancy brings big stress to the body, with increases of 15-50 percent demands on heart rate, amount of blood the heart pumps, respiration, and kidney function. These risks go way up as you age, and are especially high for women over forty. Being in good shape will help reduce these risks, as well as help you heal speedily and return to normal physical activities post C-section.

One night at the hospital, a nurse called me to come evaluate a woman who was postpartum day 2. "Tanesha" was forty-one years old and had been in labor with her first baby. She'd really wanted to have the baby naturally. But the baby wouldn't descend, so after pushing for nearly four hours, they had rushed her to the OR for a cesarean.

The nurse had tried to get her up out of bed to the bathroom, but Tanesha had buckled and fallen to the floor. Fortunately, the nurse was right beside her, and she eased her down so that she didn't fall and hit her head.

When I arrived, Tanesha was back in bed. On physical examination, I noticed she had weakness in bending her right knee, and mild numbness along the top of the thigh on the same side. As it turned out, her legs had been pushed back during labor—her right leg by her husband (a big guy, and over 6'2"), and her left leg by the nurse. Her birthing team had only been trying to help, but they'd actually injured her in the process!

Tanesha had some right leg muscle over-stretching, and moderate right side femoral nerve injury from the leg being pushed back and not resting in between pushes. She got anti-inflammatory medication and physical/occupational therapy to help her walk without giving in to the weakness in her leg. She went home with only a slight limp and, thanks to early recognition and proper therapy, improved over the next two weeks.

Would Tanesha have snapped right back to her old self had she been a few years younger? Maybe. Or maybe the *real* lesson to be learned is that husbands need to be very careful in their efforts to help their wives!

Rooming In

The trend in hospitals today is for you to have your baby with you as much as possible, also called "rooming in." This allows you to have more time to bond with your baby, breastfeed if you so choose, and enjoy your little bundle of joy.

However, if you have had a difficult birthing experience—i.e., you've gone through labor, pushed for three hours, and then wound up with a cesarean—you will probably be pretty wiped out. After some bonding with the baby, it might be wise to ask the nurse to take the baby so you can sleep. Your body heals more when you sleep then when you are being active.

And don't forget the psychological stress of having a baby, whether you labored and pushed or had an elective cesarean. You've been worried about not just your baby, but also your own health and safety. If you need some rest, get it—you're allowed. And you may need to limit your visitors, too. Have an established time for your family and friends to visit, and keep the visits short if you are tired. Be kind to yourself. After just having a baby, your deserve it!

How Long Should You Stay?

How long you stay in the hospital after your C-section depends on several factors—what shape you were in pre-operatively, how you are doing now, and how strong you feel. Hospitals send women home anywhere between two and four days after cesarean deliveries, though two days is a bit fast for most women. The insurance companies only used to cover two days in the hospital after cesarean. Then, in a presumed backlash, California passed a law that insurance had to cover for up to four days. This varies from state to state.

It's really up to you how long you want to stay. The decision may also depend on how much help you are going to be getting at home, and how much responsibility you have awaiting you—like other small children who want your attention, too. Some women like to stay in the hospital for as long as they can. Why not have the extra help?

If you are doing well, there is little reason to stay for the fourth day . . . unless you just love the hospital food, of course. Many women like the comfort of their own bed and familiar surroundings. And of course, at home, no one is coming into your room to take your blood pressure, ask questions, and change your routine every couple of hours.

I've seen women on both ends of the spectrum—those who struggle through slow and arduous recoveries, and those who recover remarkably fast. So much of it has to do with you—what kind of shape you're in, the ways you've prepared, and your mental attitude.

Take "Claire," a woman who was in labor for three days, pushed for three hours, and then wound up with a cesarean. Claire was a larger woman; she'd always struggled with her weight, and during her pregnancy, she indulged in most (if not all) of her pregnancy urges. She ate a lot of sugary foods with a high glycemic index and even developed diabetes during her second trimester.

Having double the physical stress on her body, Claire needed extra pain medication after her C-section. But she didn't take it. She could barely move around, yet she was adamant about not taking too many medicines—she would tough it out. On postpartum day 2 she could hardly walk; she was bent over and shuffling like a woman thirty years her senior.

Claire eventually caved and took extra pain medicine, but she had to stay an extra day in the hospital. Going home wasn't much better; she took weeks to get back to some basic daily activities without discomfort.

Now contrast Claire's tale with the following story. "Penny" was in her mid-thirties and was in excellent shape, both physically and mentally. Her body was strong, fortified by a moderate daily exercise routine of swimming and yoga. She also began doing Kegel exercises to get her pelvic floor muscles fired up and in shape. Penny ate almost exclusively organic foods and adhered to a strict regimen of prenatal vitamins, probiotics, and fish oil during her pregnancy.

Penny read up on different delivery options, doing extensive research on which method would be best for her and her baby. After months of study, she was well-educated and well-informed, and she decided on an elective cesarean. Her surgery went off without a hitch, and she went home after two days in the hospital. She felt fine and had her pain under control with oral medications. She knew there was nothing the hospital could provide that she could not do herself at home. Penny had quieted her fears of pregnancy and blazed forth, calm and confident.

The better you prepare yourself—both physically and psychologically—the faster you, too, will heal.

* * *

After two to four days, you'll be packing up and heading out of the hospital with baby in tow. You've escaped the beeping monitors and bad Jell-O, but recovery isn't over yet. Now let's talk about what to do once you've arrived at home, sweet home.

Things To Keep In Mind

- The more you know, the calmer, the more smoothly and faster your recovery will be. So you can focus on what's really important—your baby!

- Once you can have fluids, go slow! Start with little sips of non-sugared drinks.

- Breastfeeding will actually help you lose pregnancy weight faster.

- If you are having trouble, ask for a lactation consultation.

- Moving around will also help prevent you from getting a pulmonary embolism or deep vein thrombosis.

- Your body will start to "mobilize" the fluid in your tissues on its own, urinating it all out in one or two days, and may take a couple of weeks to return to normal.

- Take your pain medicines—women who experience more pain right after delivery had more pain chronically—one year later!

- Taking your vitamins helps you and your child, through your breast milk.

- By far the most common mainstay of pain relief after a C-section is epidural or spinal morphine.

- Alternative pain therapies are also a possibility, though they're not widely available in the USA. These include acupuncture, TENS, biofeedback, hypnosis, or EFT.

- Regular headaches are common postpartum.

- If you have diabetes, remain vigilant and maintain tight control of your blood sugar after you deliver.

- More and more women are waiting until later in life to have children. If you are an older mother, be sure to be in great cardiovascular shape.

- The trend in hospitals today is for you to have your baby with you as much as possible, also called "rooming in." This allows you to have more time to bond with your baby, breastfeed if you so choose, and enjoy your little bundle of joy.

- It's really up to you how long you want to stay in the hospital after your C-section. Many women leave on the third day after their c-section if things are going well.

Go to www.SafeBabySystem.com/bonus for additional information.

REFERENCES

[i] Birch EE. Am J Clin Nutr 2010;91:848–59. The DIAMOND (DHA Intake And Measurement Of Neural Development) Study: a double-masked, randomized controlled clinical trial of the maturation of infant visual acuity as a function of the dietary level of docosahexaenoic acid.

[ii] Minns LM. Prostaglandins Leukot Essent Fatty Acids. 2010 Apr-Jun;82(4-6):287-93. Epub 2010 Mar 5.Toddler formula supplemented with docosahexaenoic acid (DHA) improves DHA status and respiratory health in a randomized, double-blind, controlled trial of US children less than 3 years of age.

[iii] Mitchell T. Surgery Vitamins new research finding confirm previous studies showing that healing can be accelerated with proper nutrition. Life Extension Foundation Sept 1999.

[iv] Vaxman F et al. Can the would healing process be improved by vitamin supplementation? Experimental study on humans. Eur Surg Res. 1996:28:306-14.

[v] Choi BS et al. Effect of coenzyme Q10 on cutaneous healing in skin-incised mice. Arch Pharm Res. 2009 Jun;32(6):907-13.

[vi] Kainu JP et al. Persistent pain after caesarean section and vaginal birth: a cohort study. Int J OBstet Anesthesia 2010:19:4-9.

[vii] Sng BL. Incidence and risk factors for chronic pain after caesarean section under spinal anaesthesia. Anaesth Intensive Care 2009:37:748-52.

[viii] Zakowski MI. Postoperative complications associated with regional anesthesia in the parturient. In Obstetric Anesthesia, 2nd edition. Edited by Norris M, Lippincott Williams & Wilkins, Philadelphia, 1999.

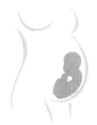

Chapter 10

Home Sweet Home

Welcome home! Now that you're back, the real recovery begins. Above all else, remember not to rush it. No matter how great you feel and how excited you are to bring your new baby home, you'll still need to take it easy for quite a while.

Your full physical, mental, and emotional recovery is very important, not just to you, but also to your new family—your husband or partner, any older children you may have, and your new baby in particular. You need to recover quickly and completely so that you can be at your best.

Your OB will probably tell you that it takes six weeks to recovery. That's the standard advice—don't lift or strain for six weeks. Obviously, your activity level will depend on what kind of shape you were in before your cesarean, nutrition level, psychological well-being, and your knowledge of how to cope with postpartum stresses. Since you're reading this book, you've already got that last one in the bag!

Many women I've spoken to say it took them significantly longer than six weeks until they really felt back to normal. Others have told me that they bounced back relatively quickly. What are the differences between the two? And how can you make sure you fall into the second camp?

Fortunately, there are many things you can do to help your recovery and minimize pain. In this chapter, I'll share with you many tips and strategies, and all the easy little things you can do to help yourself heal.

Around the House

Remember the tip about holding your scar when moving around the postpartum room? The same rule applies once you're at home. Any time you move, make sure to apply pressure against your incisional area. By providing counter force in the area where your surgery was, you'll decrease any pain you may feel.

Many women ask me how soon they can get back to regular activity. Well, not as fast as you would probably like. Remember: having a C-section is different from having a baby vaginally—it's real surgery. They open you up, move your bladder, and fiddle with your insides. The point being, don't expect your body to act like nothing happened. You have to give your body a chance to heal with time, and to take smart baby steps until you get there.

Be extra careful during the weeks following your C-section. Normal household activities—leaning, stooping, sitting in front of the computer—can be quite painful if attempted the wrong way. Don't carry or lift *anything* for at least two weeks. Then, if you are doing well, try lifting light items—less than 20 pounds (10 kilograms). If it hurts, then wait another week. The standard doctor line is not to do anything physical—lifting, straining, physical activity (including sex)—for six weeks. Most women don't wait that long, while others hurt even after six weeks. Just take it easy, and gradually test yourself to see how you're holding up.

When you *are* ready to start lifting again, remember to stand and lift with your legs, not your back. Be sure to use the right muscles. Your thighs and buttocks are the major muscle groups in your body, and they're much stronger than the back muscles. Hopefully you worked on strengthening your core abdominal muscles during pregnancy; these muscles help stabilize your back and body and provide the proper support for most everything you do.

As soon as you can, you should start some simple, low-stress exercises. The faster you get back to exercising, the stronger you become, and the faster you'll get to full recovery. Start with something easy. Just walk around. Lie on a yoga mat and do some simple stretches. A professional trainer's suggestion: Better to move in and out of a stretch than to hold it. The hormone "relaxin" of pregnancy and post-partum can allow you to overstretch things a bit. If it hurts, don't push it. Remember that the more you move around, the more you mobilize fluid, and the more your muscles and joints return to normal. The sooner that happens, the faster you'll feel yourself returning to your pre-pregnancy status.

Many women get so consumed by taking care of their new baby that they forget to take care of themselves. Don't let this happen to you! You need to take naps, stay well-hydrated, have some adult time with friends, and yes—even escape for an hour or two. It's more than okay to ask for help from friends and family; in fact it's important for your health and sanity that you do. Don't underestimate the need for some help when you first get home from the hospital. Remember that by taking care of yourself first, you'll be better able to take care of others. And there's no harm in reminding your spouse or partner that the occasional massage helps, too!

INSIDER SECRET

Even after you're pretty much back to normal, there are some tricks to reduce scar formation. Some popular over-the-counter medications are available to rub into the scar. Old remedies include vitamin E and cocoa butter. Many drugstores sell patches that contain silicone, which has also been shown to help. Other ways include laser or surgical scar revision. If you have a history of excessive scar formation, called keloids, some OBs will inject a steroid into the skin as they are closing it to help you heal.

Like we discussed in Chapter 9, you also want to make sure you are taking a good quality multivitamin to help you build new connective tissue to heal your wounds. A recent study showed that vitamin C (also called ascorbic acid) stimulated more collagen fibers and had anti-inflammatory and healing effects, providing a good environment for faster skin repair.[i] So don't forget your vitamin C!

You can also help your body to recover by giving it the building blocks it needs to replace what was lost. That includes improving your red blood cells, which carry oxygen to your tissues, and your white blood cells, which fight infection. Nutrients that help rebuild your red blood cell count include iron, folate, vitamin B6, and vitamin B12. You can help your white cells function effectively by avoiding toxins and having good nutrition, including taking vitamins and zinc.

So you're taking your vitamins and you're doing your exercises. Now what about those other "extracurriculars"? Some moms and dads probably want to know when their *personal* physical activities can return to normal. Again, the standard advice is to wait six weeks until everything is typically healed. But beware: sometimes pelvic pain can occur with intercourse.

The good news is that a C-section will probably interrupt your sex life less than if you delivered naturally. In one study, sexual intercourse aggravated pain significantly less after a cesarean than a vaginal delivery.[ii] However, even one year after birth, 23 percent of women reported that sex was painful.[iii] When it comes to making love, use common sense.

Fighting Infection

If you thought you were out of the danger zone of infection after leaving the hospital, think again. Even once you're safely ensconced in your own home, you have to be on the lookout for bleeding, pain, and signs of infection. When you leave the hospital, they'll give you instructions on what to look for and a list of common problems. But just to be extra safe, we're going to go over some precautions now.

Infections can still develop at the superficial skin site, deeper within the uterus, or even from breastfeeding. Check your incision site daily for the first week or two. The skin should appear normal, without drainage or redness. If the skin is red, hardened, smells bad, or is leaking fluid other than a small amount of clear fluid, you should call your OB right away. Those are all potential signs of infections.

You should also be checking how much vaginal fluid is coming out (called discharge). Some fluid is to be expected and is entirely normal, like a heavy menstruation, for several weeks. Again, pay close attention to whether it is clear or discolored (yellow or green), smells foul, looks like blood (red is fresh blood, brown is old blood). Pain and fever are also signs of infection.

Here are two other common infections that many women develop during their postpartum weeks:

Urinary Tract Infections

We've yet to talk about urinary tract infections, one of the most common infections that women develop. A UTI may develop from having had a Foley catheter placed during your cesarean (the prophylactic antibiotics typically given during surgery may suppress infection until later). Signs of a UTI include frequent urination, discoloration, foul smell, pain with urination, pain in your back (indicates kidney infection), fever, blood in your urine, and an increase in your white blood cell count. If you think you might have a urinary tract infection, call your OB.

Mastitis

Mastitis is an infection in the breast from feeding that afflicts many new mothers. Fever, pain, redness,

> **INSIDER SECRET**
>
> You can prevent cracked nipples by washing your nipples with warm water (*never* use soap) after every feeding

and hardness are all signs of breast infection. Typically mastitis starts with dry, cracked nipples, so make sure to keep them moisturized with vitamin E, olive oil, or another preferred moisturizer, like pure lanolin.

Hopefully you were taking good bacteria during your pregnancy. You can (and should) continue to take probiotics after your delivery, too. By having the good bacteria colonized along your gastrointestinal tract and vagina, you can help prevent infection. Endometritus, infection of the uterus, occurs in 8.6 percent of women post-operatively, and the majority of uterine infections come from bacteria in the vagina and cervix.[iv] Another study showed that endometritus was decreased when women were taking probiotics.[v] Beating bad bacteria with good bacteria—how cool is that?

Keeping Pain in Check

Your doctor will give you a prescription for pain medicines when you get home. If you are having significant pain, you should let your OB know. As long as the pain doesn't signify something more serious, you should be able to adequately treat it.

Pain has been noted to be woefully undertreated in the USA, and the postpartum period is a prime example. Most doctors are not trained as pain specialists the way anesthesiologists are. So let me give you a few tips that they may unintentionally forget to give you. First and foremost: treat the pain well!

As we discussed in the last chapter, the net result of taking pain medication is that you will recover faster. Since pain is to a large extent learned, "toughing it out" doesn't make physiological sense. Post-cesarean pain should not be severe for more than one week; you won't get addicted in that time frame. After that, you should be able to cut back on medication. Taking strong narcotics beyond one week could mean you need to be reevaluated, and you should be weaning yourself off the drugs before then.

By taking your pain medicine, you will be more comfortable, enjoy and bond with your baby, and be able to move around more. The studies are conclusive: if you have severe pain immediately after your cesarean, you are more likely to develop chronic pain down the line.[vii] Pain medicine will help you move around and do your routine: the perfect launching pad to a complete recovery.

You can lower the kind of narcotic you need by taking more than one kind of medicine—called multi-modal analgesia. If you have significant pain, you want to combine some narcotic and an anti-inflammatory like ibuprofen. By attacking the pain by two different pathways, the pain relief will be better. And remember to stagger your medications; always take them at least two hours apart. This will ensure that they peak and wear off at different times, leading to continuous relief and a smoother ride.

> **INSIDER SECRET**
>
> Most doctors prefer to prescribe Vicodin over Percocet, but not for the reason you may think. Because Percocet is a schedule II drug, it means there's higher potential for abuse, and the government tracks prescriptions for it. That means more hassle for your OB.

The most common strong pain medicine prescribed is Vicodin (hydrocodone and acetaminophen), a DEA Schedule III drug. A few doctors will give a stronger painkiller, commonly known as Percocet (oxycodone and acetaminophen), a DEA Schedule II drug. If you're having a lot of pain when you get home and the Vicodin isn't cutting it, just know that you don't have to suffer; there are stronger pain medicines available.

Many women complain to me that they don't like taking Vicodin; either it doesn't work for them or it makes them nauseous, and they prefer Percocet. There are others who feel the exact opposite. The point is that if one pain medicine doesn't do it for you, you can try the other. Just expect a bit more red tape if you need the Percocet.

Tylenol with Codeine is also a mid-level pain reliever and is a Schedule III drug. Tylenol with codeine is generally considered not quite as strong as Vicodin at the typical dose, but remains an excellent choice.

Your pain relief will be most effective if you pair your choice of narcotic with your favorite over-the-counter non-steroidal anti-inflammatory drug (NSAID) like ibuprofen or naproxen. You probably know which one agrees with you better. People with bleeding problems or gastrointestinal ulcers may be advised not to take them.

Shockingly, women who have cesareans have a significant chance of developing chronic pain (pain lasting longer than six months). While most women recover from a cesarean in the official six weeks, many women take longer, with at least 10 percent developing chronic pain and 10 percent developing postpartum depression.[viii] In another study, 36 percent of women had pain two months after cesarean, and 10-18 percent still had pain one year later.[ix]

INSIDER SECRET

Chronic pain from cesareans. While 36 percent of women had pain two months after cesarean, a whopping 10-18 percent still had pain one year later. Take your pain medicines early to reduce spinal cord 'wind up' and chronic pain later.

The absolute best way to help reduce your chance of chronic pain is to utilize preemptive analgesia. Treat the pain before it starts so that your spinal cord never has the chance to become sensitized to it. In other words, avoiding pain in the short term prevents pain in the long term. It's like having your cake and eating it too!

Of course there's always the fine print. The dark side of narcotics is that the same receptors that take away pain also slow the gastrointestinal tract motility. In layman's terms? Any narcotic can give you constipation. If you get constipated, you can bloat, have abdominal pain, and need more pain medications. The pain medications you get from your OB are typically safe for breast-feeding, but be sure to ask.

Remember to drink lots of water, especially if you are breastfeeding. Being well-hydrated will be good for your stool regularity and softness. Taking your probiotics will increase the bulk and softness of your stools, too. And don't forget the fiber. You might also need a stool softener like Colace. Or you can take magnesium citrate, which helps constipation and has the added benefit of upping your magnesium levels, a mineral in which many people are chronically low.

A Healthy Mom is a Happy Mom

We've covered all the ways to enhance and expedite your physical recovery—exercising, taking vitamins, reducing your pain, and going easy on yourself. But what about taking care of yourself on the *inside*?

Having a C-section doesn't just take a toll on your body; it is emotionally draining as well. Your hormones have been swinging wildly, you're sleep-deprived, and if you're a new parent, you're probably on an emotional roller coaster. Your partner feels ignored and you've already forgotten what life was like before you had a baby.

One of your top priorities is to actively seek out ways to minimize stress and anxiety. Learn to quiet the fears of pregnancy. When stress takes over, your body actually fights its natural impulse, which is to heal. Your body wants to do its thing and repair itself; it's only your mind that's getting in the way. Just imagine yourself recovering, and let your body take over from there. It knows exactly what to do.

Of course your mental and emotional well-being are intimately related to your physical condition. Getting adequate sleep, eating nutritiously wholesome food, taking fish oil, and exercising will all contribute to your peace of mind. Meditation and quiet time also help to maintain balance. Hypnosis audios, Eastern techniques such as Chi Qong, and EFT have been helpful to many women as well. See www.SafeBabySystem.com for some helpful tips about these and other remedies.

INSIDER SECRET

Postpartum depression strikes 1 in 9 women. Pain after giving birth and depression have been linked. Take your pain meds and be alert for signs of depression: tired all the time, feeling inexplicably sad, excessive crying, a lack of energy or motivation, eating too much or too little. If you experience any of these, Seek professional help

Sometimes even these resources are not enough. It's important that you recognize when you're not doing well emotionally, and to have the courage to ask for help. When physical ailments strike, most women are able to ask for help, especially if it involves pain or not being able to perform daily activities. However, many women (and men!) have trouble recognizing and seeking help for emotional ailments.

Postpartum depression occurs in 5-10 percent of women. One study found pain and depression to be linked, with 11 percent of women showing signs of depression eight weeks after giving birth.[x] The signs of postpartum depression include being tired all the time, feeling inexplicably sad, excessive crying, a lack of energy or motivation, eating too much or too little, sleeping too much or too little, headaches, chest pains, sluggishness, heart palpitations, poor self-image, a decreased interest in activities you used to love, and an inability to focus or make decisions. If any of these symptoms describe you, tell your partner and seek professional help. You can't recover fast from a cesarean if you are depressed!

What causes postpartum depression? There are many different factors that precipitate it, including the sudden hormonal swings in pregnancy and childbirth, pituitary/glandular problems after delivery, and an imbalance of certain neurotransmitters in the brain. Some studies have suggested that taking fish oil can help decrease your chance for postpartum depression.[xi] Genetic variation in metabolism plays a role[xii] and low DHA in the brain has been shown to decrease serotonin levels (serotonin elevates mood).[xiii]

It's important to keep your brain's neuro-chemical transmitters in balance, including serotonin, noradrenalin, acetylcholine, and dopamine. Certain foods and nutritional supplements can provide a natural boost. Medications can also up your levels; mild anti-depressants are commonly prescribed in the U.S. during and after pregnancy (if you're breastfeeding, just be sure that the medicine won't cause potential harm to your baby). Unfortunately, however, the stigma regarding mental health persists. While 10 percent of postpartum moms meet the criteria for depression, only 1 in 5 of those women are undergoing treatment.[xiv]

You undoubtedly want to be able to be fully there for your baby, and that means being in tip-top emotional condition. If you're depressed, get help! There's no need to feel guilty or ashamed. Yes, motherhood is a wonderful thing, but it can also be scary and overwhelming. If your depression has lasted more than a few weeks, talk to your OB or midwife. They may be able to refer you to a mental health professional. It can also be helpful to attend support groups for new moms. Knowing you're not alone can make a world of difference.

Despite the new little person in your life, remember to take care of yourself and be aware of your own needs. Rest as often as you can, and ask for help when you need it. If it helps, get out of the house and away from the baby. You're still your own person—you're entitled to your own life.

And, ironically, the more you take care of yourself, the better you'll be able to take care of your baby. Don't feel guilty—it's good for both of you! When you're depressed, you aren't able to give your baby all he or she needs. So by taking time to take care of yourself, you're being the best mom you could possibly be.

> **INSIDER SECRET**
>
> Take care of yourself. Many women devote themselves to their newborn and neglect themselves. The more you take care of yourself, the better you'll be able to care for your baby. Don't feel guilty—it's good for both of you.

It's also important not to neglect the other relationships in your life. Like it or not, your relationships with your partner, other children, family, and friends are all going to change. Although you naturally deserve the lion's share of the attention and help, remember that any relationship is a two-way street. Be nice to your spouse, too! It's *always* difficult for us men to truly understand what a woman needs, but that's even more true if that woman is a new mother.

Husbands are usually equally inept with their first child, myself included. Go easy on us, and we'll do the best we can to help. If you tell us what to do, we'll do it!

If you have other children, the dynamic will obvious change. Sometimes siblings will feel confusion or even resentment at the new screeching addition to the family. One suggestion is to bring a present from the new baby to the other siblings. A simple gift can start the relationship off with some good will.

* * *

Take a long, well-deserved sigh of relief (while holding your incision, of course)—you made it! You survived a C-section, and you've got a beautiful baby to show for it. Well done, mom!

I always love to hear from mothers, so please send us your cesarean stories and how *C-Section* has helped you. Visit www.SafeBabySystem.com or email me at DrMark@SafeBabySystem.com. Help me write the next book—Send me questions and topics you would like to have answered, and I'll try to include and answer them in the next book!

I hope this book has come in handy during one of the greatest adventures of all time. Now go enjoy the new life you've brought into the world!

Things To Keep In Mind

- The real recovery begins when you return home.

- Don't lift or strain for six weeks.

- Any time you move, make sure to apply pressure against your incisional area.

- During the first weeks after your C-section, normal household activities—leaning, stooping, sitting in front of the computer—can be quite painful if attempted the wrong way.

- If you take care of yourself first, you'll be better able to take care of others. And there's no harm in reminding your spouse or partner that the occasional massage helps, too!

- The good news is that a C-section will probably interrupt your sex life less than if you delivered naturally.

- You should also be checking how much vaginal fluid is coming out (called discharge).

- Take your pain medicine—it is important to treat your pain. Acute pain can contribute to Chronic pain.

- Remember to drink lots of water, especially if you are breastfeeding.

- Getting adequate sleep, eating nutritiously wholesome food, taking fish oil, and exercising will all contribute to your peace of mind.

- If you're depressed, get help! There's no need to feel guilty or ashamed.

- Husbands are usually equally inept with their first child, myself included. Go easy on us, and we'll do the best we can to help. If you tell us what to do, we'll do it!

Go to www.SafeBabySystem.com/bonus for additional information.

REFERENCES

[i] Lima CC et al. Ascorbic acid for the healing of skin wounds in rats. Braz J Biol. 2009 Nov;69(4):1195-201.

[ii] Kainu JP et al. Persistent pain after caesarean section and vaginal birth: a cohort study. Int J OBstet Anesthesia 2010:19:4-9.

[iii] Kainu JP et al. Persistent pain after caesarean section and vaginal birth: a cohort study. Int J OBstet Anesthesia 2010:19:4-9.

[iv] Landon, M. Chapter 19 Cesarean Delivery. in Gabbe: Obstetrics: normal and problem pregnancies, 5th Ed. Edited by Gabbe S, Niebyl J, Simpson J. Churchill Livingstone Philadelphia 2007, p486-520.

[v] Marrazzo JM. Evolving issues in understanding and treating bacterial vaginosis. Expert Review of Antiinfective Therapy 2004;2: 913–22.

[vi] Eisenach JC. Severity of acute pain after childbirth, but not type of delivery, predicts persistent pain and postpartum depression. Pain 2008:140:87-94.

[vii] Eisenach JC. Severity of acute pain after childbirth, but not type of delivery, predicts persistent pain and postpartum depression. Pain 2008:140:87-94. And Lavand'homme P. Editorial. Chronic pain after vaginal and cesarean delivery: a reality questioning our daily practice of obstetric anesthesia. Int J Obstet Anesth 2010:19:1-2.

[viii] Eisenach JC. Severity of acute pain after childbirth, but not type of delivery, predicts persistent pain and postpartum depression. Pain 2008:140:87-94.

[ix] Kainu JP et al. Persistent pain after caesarean section and vaginal birth: a cohort study. Int J OBstet Anesthesia 2010:19:4-9.

[x] Eisenach JC. Severity of acute pain after childbirth, but not type of delivery, predicts persistent pain and postpartum depression. Pain 2008:140:87-94.

[xi] Makrides M. Asia Pac J Clin Nutr. 2003;12 Suppl:S37. Docosahexaenoic acid and post-partum depression - is there a link?

[xii] Xie L. J Nutrigenet Nutrigenomics. 2009;2(4-5):243-50. Epub 2010 Apr 15. Association of fatty acid desaturase gene polymorphisms with blood lipid essential fatty acids and perinatal depression among Canadian women: a pilot study.

[xiii] Levant B. *Psychoneuroendocrinology.* 2008 October; 33(9): 1279–1292. doi:10.1016/ j.psyneuen.2008.06.012. Decreased Brain Docosahexaenoic Acid Content Produces Neurobiological Effects Associated With Depression: Interactions With Reproductive Status In Female Rats.

[xiv] Marcus SM. Depression during pregnancy: rates, risks and consequences—Motherisk Update 2008. Can J Clin Pharmacol. 2009 Winter;16(1):e15-22. Epub 2009 Jan 22.

About the Author

Dr. Mark Zakowski has been Chief of Obstetric Anesthesiology for over 18 years at nationally recognized hospitals in New York City and California. **During that time, Dr. Mark has personally assisted over 24,000 women in giving birth and has been in charge of over 115,000 deliveries**, giving him unique and valuable insights on how to best ensure a happy mom, a healthy baby, and a safe delivery.

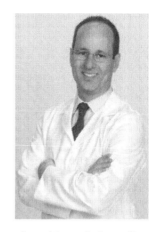

Dr. Mark has served on various departmental and hospital quality improvement committees including the **Board of Directors for the National Society of Obstetric Anesthesia and Perinatology** and **the California Society of Anesthesiologists.** He has published nearly 30 technical papers on anesthesiology and pregnancy and 38 abstracts related to birthing and anesthesiology. Dr. Mark has also has authored chapters in major Obstetric Anesthesia textbooks and been cited or provided additional material in a number of professional books related to postoperative care, critical care, and anesthesiology.

Dr. Mark received a B.S. with distinction in Biology from Stanford University and an M.D. from Albert Einstein College of Medicine. He has served as Assistant Professor, Dept. of Anesthesiology at New York University Medical Center and currently serves as Adjunct Associate Professor at a nationally prominent medical center in California.

Dr. Mark is dedicated to **quieting the fears of pregnancy and delivery.** He is the author of *C-Section: How to Avoid, Prepare for and Recover From Your Cesarean* and *The Safe Baby System* (due out in 2011).

www.SafeBabySystem.com/SafeBabyReport

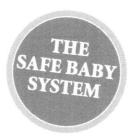

Simple Things You Can Do to Help Ensure a Problem-Free Delivery
by
Mark Zakowski, M.D.

Author, *C-Section: How to Avoid,*
Prepare for and Recover from Your Cesarean

Pregnant? Congratulations! Now is the time to get the information you need to help you have a safe pregnancy and deliver a healthy baby... with **The Safe Baby System by Dr. Mark Zakowski.**

Dr. Mark has personally **assisted over 24,000 women in giving birth,** allowing him to develop unique and valuable insights on how to best ensure a happy mom, a healthy baby, and a safe delivery. As **Chief of Obstetric Anesthesiology** for over 18 years at nationally recognized hospitals in New York City and California, **he has been in charge of more than 115,000 deliveries** — more babies than the entire population of Berkeley, California.

Dr. Mark developed **The Safe Baby System** based upon his extensive hands-on knowledge of what worked and what didn't to bring about a positive birth experience.

In **The Safe Baby System**, you will learn:

- How to help preserve your health while having a safe delivery.
- The single biggest risk to infant health… and how you can avoid it.
- Irreversible damage — and how surprisingly simple it can be to prevent it.
- The great responsibility shift: How to make certain you are prepared.
- What you can do to give your baby the best possible start in life.

Written in Dr. Mark's clear, easy-to-understand style, filled with useful tips that range from helpful to potentially life-saving, **The Safe Baby System** walks you through your pregnancy and delivery with warmth, compassion, and information you can trust.

The Safe Baby System will publish in late 2011… but you don't have to wait to learn one of Dr. Mark's most important pregnancy tips in this **Free Special Report**:

"The #1 Doctor-Approved Secret to Help Avoid the Dangers of Giving Birth to a Premature Baby While Protecting the Health of Pregnant Women"

Learn this one simple, inexpensive step you can take to protect the health of both you and the baby. **To receive this potentially life-saving information, go to:**

www.SafeBabySystem.com/SafeBabyReport

NOTES

NOTES

NOTES

16708575R00104

Made in the USA
Charleston, SC
06 January 2013